The Ultimate In-Home Golf Fitness Program

Your 12-Week Plan Towards Increased Distance, Durability, and Flexibility

Brandon Gaydorus

M.S., CSCS, PGA, TPI-2, PN-1

ISBN-13: 978-1-7932-6062-8

DEDICATION

This book is dedicated to all of the amazing people who have helped me out in various different ways over the years. Thank you.

TABLE OF CONTENTS

Chapter 1: Introduction

WHAT is this Book...

This book was designed to help golfers understand the concepts of golf fitness and to give guidance on a 12-week progressive program designed to help golfers increase distance, durability, and flexibility. In return this will give golfers the potential to improve their golf game and help prevent injuries.

WHY Am I Writing this Book...

This book exists to provide golfers with a program that they can act on, to then give them the potential to lower their scores. The information in this book has been put together from years of experience playing golf, learning from some of the top golf fitness professionals, and through training hundreds of golfers. The goal of "The Ultimate In-Home Golf Fitness Program" is to help golfers move better, feel better, and play better.

WHO Am I...

Instead of writing up the typical about me section. I want to share with you what I believe, about golf fitness to help get a better understanding of why this book was written and why this program will work...

- I believe that the more you take care of your body, the more it will take care of you.
- I believe that a functional training program gives golfers the potential to improve performance.
- I believe that a progressive system will lead to greater results.
- I believe that everyone could get to where they want faster with a great coach and a progressive plan in place.

Why I Believe This...

I believe the "The Ultimate In-Home Golf Fitness Program" will give golfers greater potential to improve performance and take a more direct approach towards massive success because of the detailed plan and progressive exercises.

What Makes This Book Different...

The workout plan offers a simple and effective approach towards keeping golfers happy, healthy, and ready to win. This is developed through a progressive program that can be executed just about anywhere with limited equipment.

The People I Have Worked With...

I have worked with juniors, high schoolers, college, amateur, and professional golfers and found a way to integrate a system that works for all.

Think About This Before Starting...

Would you agree that if you could move better, feel better, and get stronger; that you would have the potential to become a better golfer?

If you said yes, then this is likely to be the right book for you. If not, then this may not be the right book for you at this time. Also, if you are not completely satisfied with this book, contact me at bgaydorus@gmail.com with a brief explanation of why you were not satisfied and I will be happy to give your thoughts into consideration for future research.

Chapter 2: Benefits of Golf Fitness

Before we dive deep into the benefits of golf fitness, ask yourself the following questions...

-**Would you agree**, that in golf the main goal is to get the ball in the hole with the lowest amount of shots possible?

-**Would you agree**, that hitting the ball farther while maintaining accuracy will give you a distinct advantage to score lower?

-**Would you agree**, that the more you take care of your body, the more it will take care of you? And that a healthier body will keep you on the golf course longer?

If you found yourself saying yes to these questions, then you would probably agree that if this book could help you increase distance, lower your scores, and keep your body healthy to be able to play injury-free then you would follow the program, right?

Well then good, because this program is designed to help you increases distance, give you the potential to lower scores, and stay injury-free. But in case you needed research-based evidence here are some studies to help explain the benefits of a fitness program designed for golfers.

Previous studies have indicated...

*That there is a direct correlation to low handicap golfers and high levels of club head speed at impact (6, 15).

*A significant increase with golfers in total or carry distance through a functional training program (4, 5, 9, 11, 12, 13).

*A significant increase in golfers in club head speed through a functional training program (10, 14).

*A significant increase in golfers ball speed through a functional training program (1).

*Training programs have improved golf performance for recreational or mid-high handicap golfers (8, 10, 13, 14) and with low handicap or professional golfers (1, 4, 5, 11, 12).

These studies show the potential benefits of a golf fitness program. But most importantly no matter what the program is, it should be designed to safely keep participants healthy, while increasing the golfer's potential to improve performance.

A typical functional training program tends to focus on movements that address an individual's flexibility, core stability, balance, and strength through resistance training (14).

- Addressing flexibility will give golfers the potential to increase range of motion in their joints.
- Increased core stability helps to improve spinal stability and spinal stability is needed to control the three variables of the trunk in the golf swing, specifically flexion/extension, lateral flexion, and axial rotation (17).
- Improving balance will help enhance neuromuscular control. Neuromuscular exercises can consist of a combination of exercises tailored around balance, strength, plyometrics, agility, and sport-specific movements (18).
- Resistance training gives individuals the potential to gain strength and power to hit the ball farther (14).

With proper strength in the hips, core, and shoulders, stability in the knees, pelvis, lumbar spine, scapulae, and elbows, and mobility in the shoulders, hips, and thoracic spine, golfers will have characteristics built in, to swing with more efficiency (16). Below is a picture of the main mobile and stable joints of the body (7).

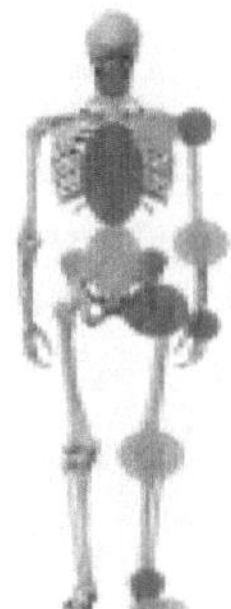

The joints that go in a circular motion are considered mobile joints and should be able to move appropriately to allow the golfer to get into the correct positions for an efficient golf swing. An example of proper mobility in relation to golf, would be if the golfer has proper range of motion in the thoracic spine, they will have an increased potential to create a full backswing and smooth transition throughout the downswing.

With adequate mobility there needs to be appropriate stability. Stability allows the joints to stay under control. With no stability the golfer would not be able to transition back into the downswing.

The stable joints typically move in one direction -- which is either side to side, forward and back, or up and down. Many stable joints do go in multiple directions but with a limited range.

Chapter 3 – Foam Rolling:

Benefits of Self-Myofascial Release include better circulation (increased blood flow) and reduced muscle soreness. A foam roller is basically a cheaper version of a massage therapist. Manual work is typically always better, but foam rolling is a practical alternative.

Each foam rolling sequence should consist of about 6-15 rolls, depending on the person and how it feels.

Outer Thigh (IT Band and TFL)

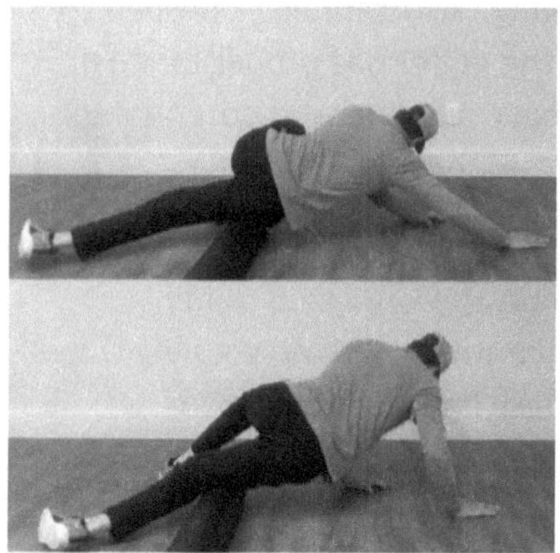

To Perform…

-Place two hands on the ground and one foot forward, this helps stabilize the body

-Proceed to roll the outside of the leg

Lower Back (Quadratus Lumborum)

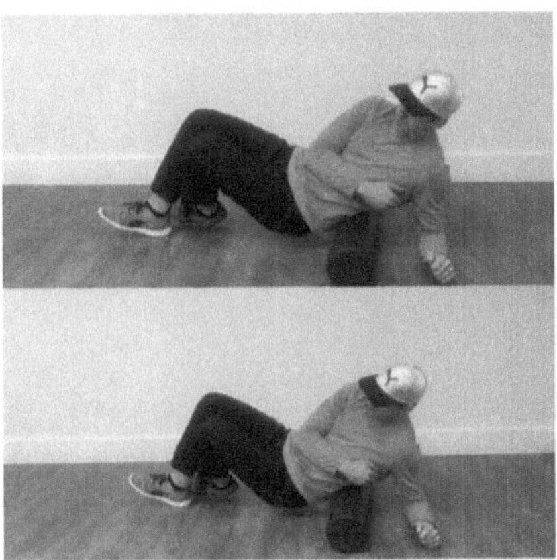

To Perform...

-Place the foam roller on the side of the low back and proceed to roll up and down

-This should be gentle from this position and the roller SHOULD NOT touch the middle of the spine

Mid-to-Upper Back (Paraspinal – Erector Spinae – Muscles)

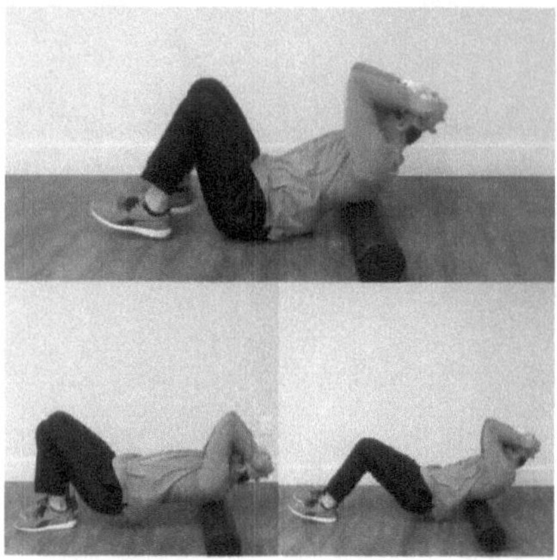

To Perform…

-Place the foam roller on the upper part of the back

-Pinch the elbows together to make sure the back is nice and tight

-Then proceed to roll the upper to middle of the back area

Back Shoulder Muscles (Latissimus Dorsi and Teres Major)

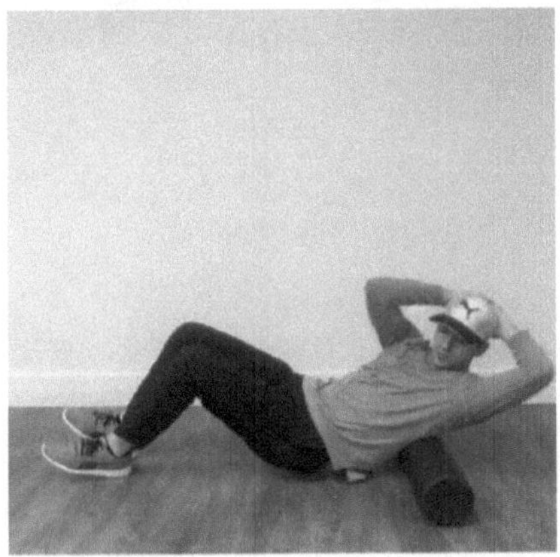

To Perform...

-Place the hands behind the head

-Proceed to roll the lat area of the back

Front of Leg (Tibialis Anterior)

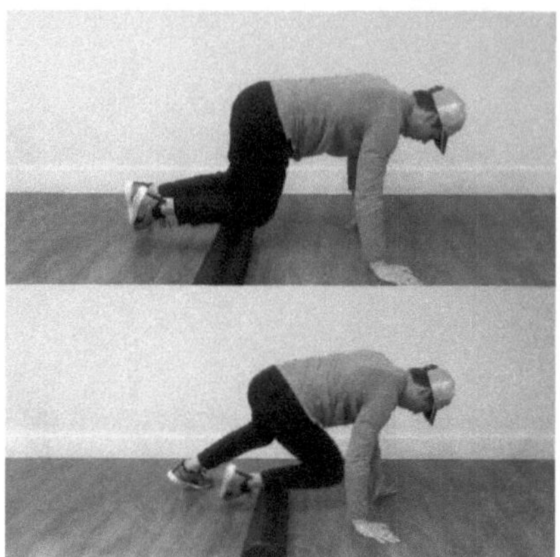

To Perform...

-Place one shin on the foam roller with the opposing foot and both hands stabilizing the body

-Proceed to roll the muscle that is located to the side of the shin (Outer Part)

Posterior (Gluteus and Piriformis)

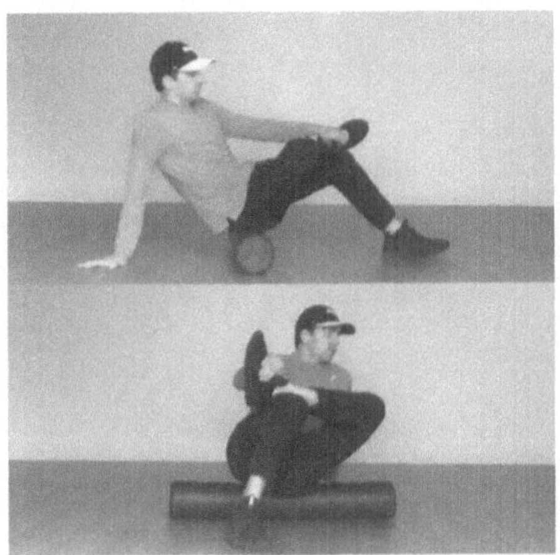

To Perform...

-Roll one glute at a time

-Place one heel on the opposite knee to help lengthen the glute

-Roll glute with the foot that is up on the knee

Back of the Thigh (Hamstrings)

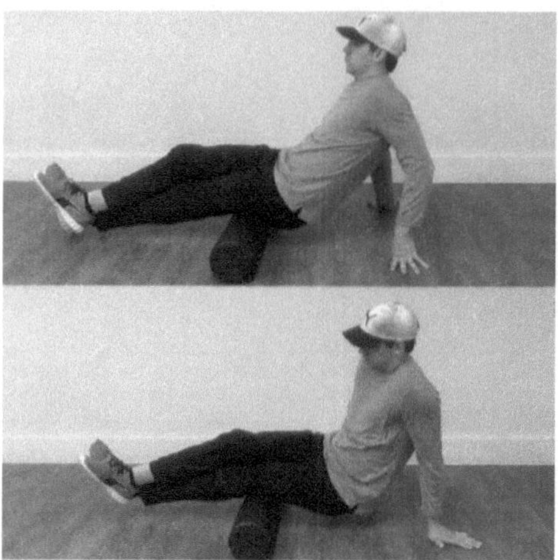

To Perform...

-Place one leg over the other and use the hands to help guide the body forward and backward

-Proceed to roll the hamstring muscles up and down

Calf (Gastrocnemius and Soleus)

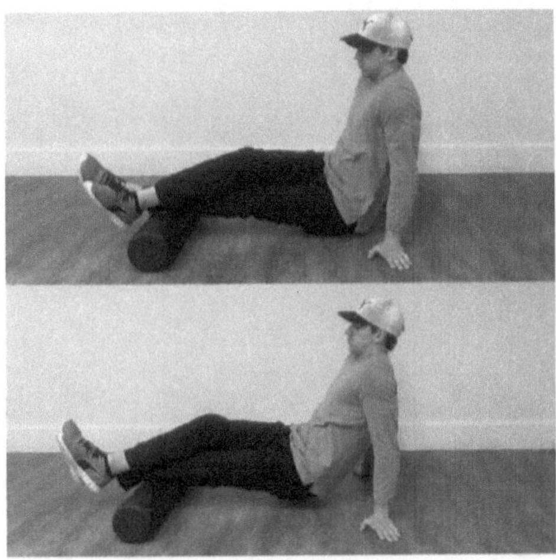

To Perform...

-Place one leg over the other and the hands on the ground to help guide the movement forward and backward

-Proceed to roll the calf

Front of Thigh Muscles (Quadriceps)

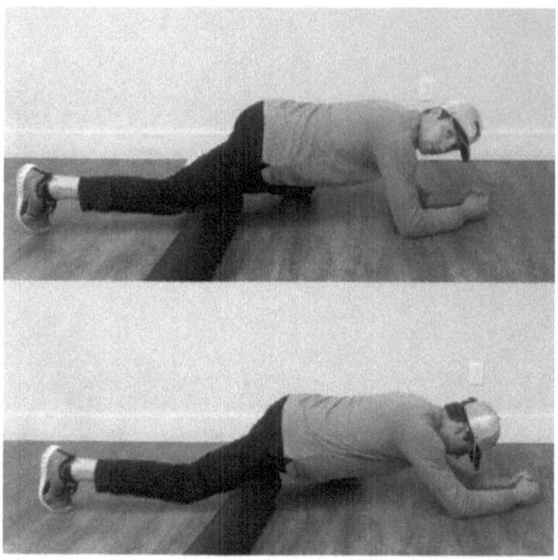

To Perform...

-Place the forearms on the ground

-Also place the outside knee and ankle on the ground to help guide the movement

-Proceed to roll out the quadricep (top half of the front part of the leg)

Inner Thigh/Groin (Adductors)

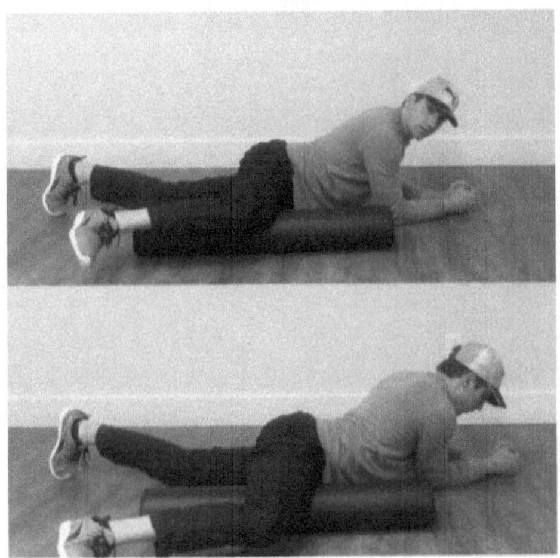

To Perform...

-Place the roller on the inside of the leg

-Try to get the leg being rolled out to form a 90-degree angle

-Roll back and forth

Biceps

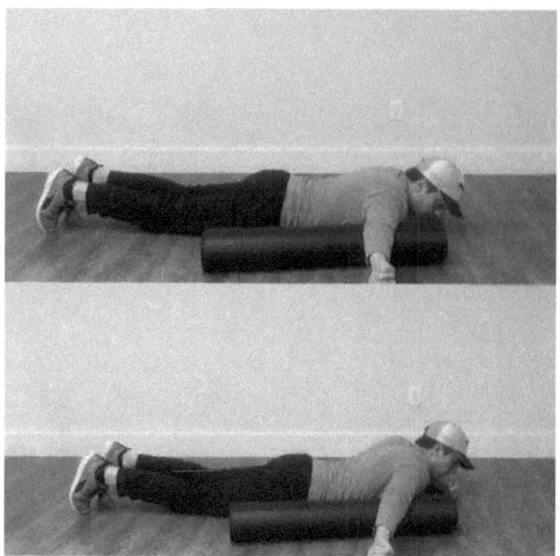

To Perform...

-Laying in the prone position (on stomach), place the bicep on the roller by reaching the arm out to the side

-Proceed to roll back and forth

Triceps

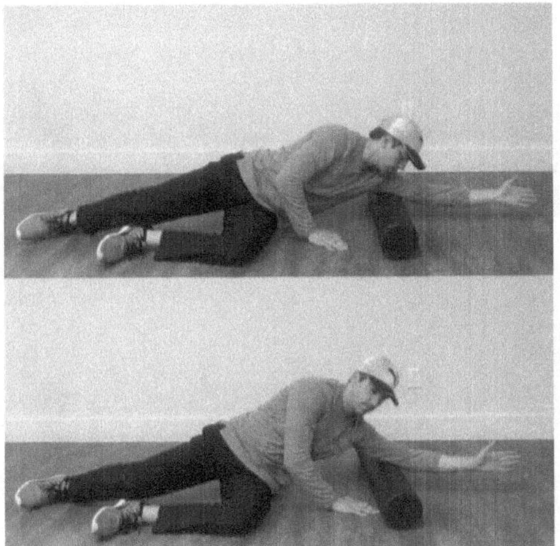

To Perform...

-Extend triceps and arm

-Proceed to roll back and forth

Back of Shoulder (Posterior Rotator Cuff)

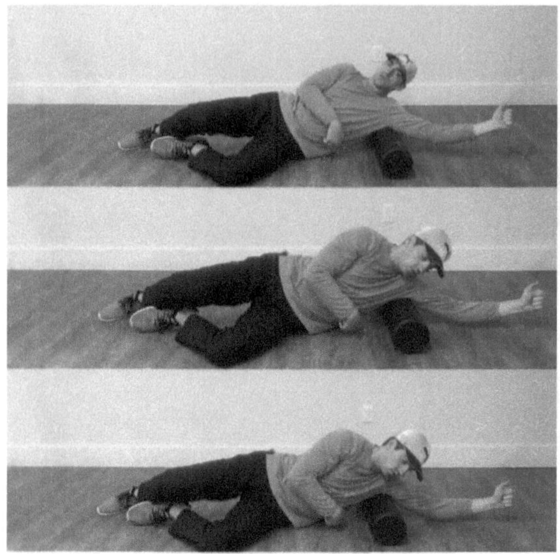

To Perform...

-Place foam roller towards the back of the armpit

-Roll side to side

Inside of Forearm (Forearm Flexors)

Outer Forearm (Forearm Extensors)

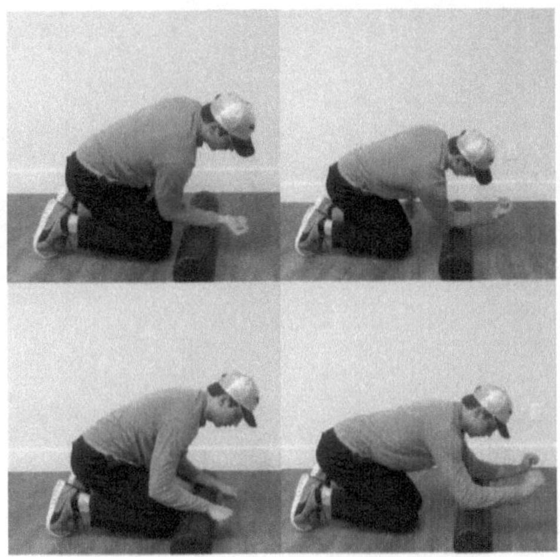

To Perform...

-Place forearms on the roller

-As the foam roller comes closer to the body reach the hands up toward the sky

Recap of Muscles to Foam Roll:

Calf (Gastrocnemius and Soleus)

Front of Leg (Tibialis Anterior)

Front of Thigh Muscles (Quadriceps)

Inner Thigh/Groin (Adductors)

Back of the Thigh (Hamstrings)

Outer Thigh (IT Band and TFL)

Posterior (Gluteus and Piriformis)

Lower Back (Quadratus Lumborum)

Mid to Upper Back (Paraspinal – Erector Spinae – Muscles)

Back of Shoulder (Posterior Rotator Cuff)

Back Shoulder Muscles (Latissimus Dorsi and Teres Major)

Inside of Your Forearm (Forearm Flexors)

Outer Forearm (Forearm Extensors)

*It is important to note that there are plenty of other muscles that can be foam rolled. These cover a basic foam rolling circuit that if done properly and consistently can be very effective.

*Also, if there is a sharp pain when foam rolling a specific area, please see a medical professional instead of trying to roll away the pain.

Chapter 4: Point of the Warm-Up

Essentially, the main goal of a warm-up is to prepare the body and mind appropriately to increase the effectiveness of the workout and help participants avoid injury.

The four secrets to an effective warm-up for golfers include:

1.) Priming the Mobility that you already have:
We brush our teeth every day to keep them looking and feeling good. Therefore, we should move our joints every day to keep them healthy and moving well.

2.) Prepare the Central Nervous System (CNS):
The CNS is made up of the brain and spinal cord.

The **brain** is an organ made up of nervous tissue that pioneers the actions and thoughts of the human body.

The **spinal cord** relays the information from the rest of the body to the brain.

With proper movement and coordination exercises built into the warm-up the central nervous system will be prepared efficiently (8).

3.) Increase Tissue Temperature:
The warm-up should warm you up, increasing the tissue temperature of the body will allow it to absorb and adapt more efficiently to the stress of the workout and/or golf round.

4.) Specific to the Task at Hand:
The most golf specific warm-up would be swinging a golf club and should be incorporated into a warm-up routine before a round of golf.

*For advice on golf swing warm-ups contact your local PGA Professional or skip to the Super Speed protocols in the conditioning section of the book. The Super Speed protocol is not only good for conditioning but also great for warming up.

Breakdown of the Phases

It is encouraged to start from the phase 1 movements and then progress accordingly.

With the 12-Week Plan it is recommended to execute each phase for 4 weeks.

For example...

Week 1-4: Phase 1

Week 5-8: Phase 2

Week 9-12: Phase 3

There are also progressions (harder) and regressions (easier) for necessary exercises to target individual needs. If the individual cannot execute the progression with efficient form, then stick with the previous phase. It is important that we move efficiently first before progressing to the more advanced exercises.

Joint-by-Joint Warm-Up

The concepts of the joint-by-joint warm-up were first brought to my attention by Gray Cook in the book "Movement" and Michael Boyle in the book "Advances in Functional Training" (2, 3). For this specific book, the warm-up is explained starting from the joints closet to the ground and then up from there.

The warm-up is simply based around preparing the body and mind for physical activity. As talked about above, preparing the body properly for a warm-up tends to lead to increased effectiveness for the workout and prepares the central nervous system for physical activity. The goal of the joint-by-joint warm-up is to move the joints the way they are meant to move, to help properly prepare the body for a progressive overload on the muscles.

Without incorporating the full joint-by-joint warm-up into your workout routine there will likely be an increased chance of injury and stiffness. With the joint-by-joint warm-up, all main joints are targeted and should be primed for an effective workout!

In this book, the joint-by-joint warm-up is designed in three different phases. The phases are designed in a manner that enforce an increase in demand of stability, to efficiently progress the joints to move properly with an effective system. For the proper progression we first start from the supinated position (lying on back), then progress to a quadruped (hands and knees)/kneeling position, and then finally to a standing position.

For the mobile joints there are both linear and lateral movements to ensure that the joints are being moved throughout their different planes of motion, while the stable joints have 1-2 exercises based on the main plane of motion that they are meant to move in.

Ankle (Mobile Joint):

Phase 1:

Linear - Supine Ankle Flexion + Extension

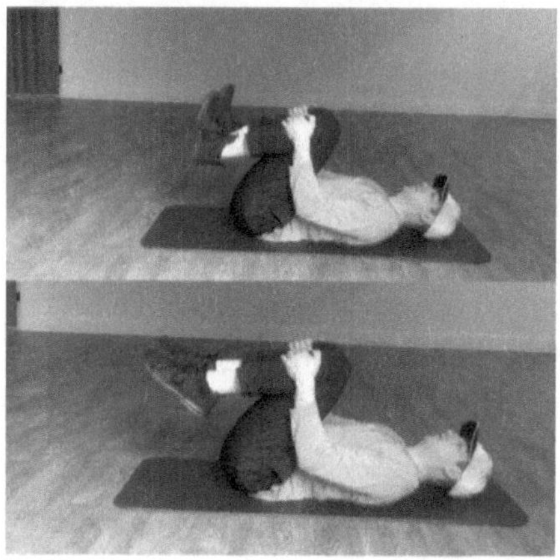

To Perform...

-Hug the knees

-Flex toes towards the knees and hold for 1 second

-Then extend toes towards the ground and hold for 1 second

Lateral – Supine Ankle Windshield Wipers

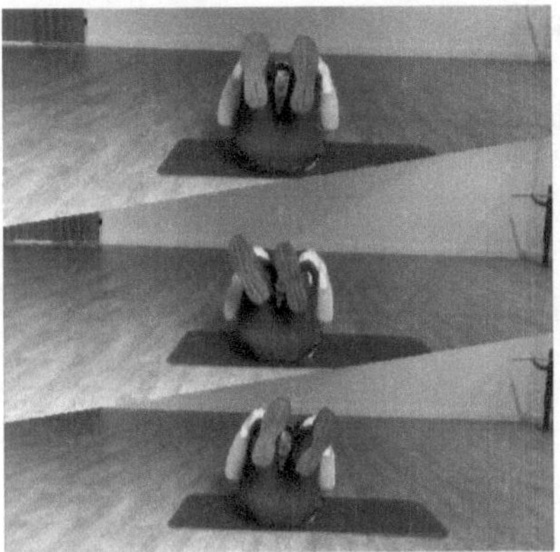

To Perform...

-Hug the knees

-Flex toes towards the knees

-Then proceed to turn the ankles side to side like a windshield wiper

Phase 2:

Linear: Half-Kneeling Ankle Dorso-Flexion

Lateral: Half-Kneeling Side to Side Ankle Dorso-Flexion

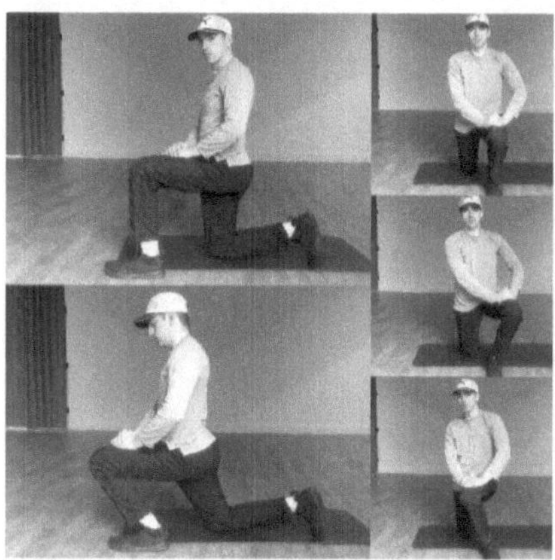

To Perform...

Half-Kneeling Ankle Dorso-Flexion

-Start from the half-kneeling position with the knee just above the ankle

-Drive the knee past the toes of the lead leg

-Use the hands to help drive the knee further forward

Half-Kneeling Side to Side Ankle Dorso-Flexion

-Proceed with the same steps from above just with the knee going forward as it goes to the left and then to the right

Phase 3:

Linear - Standing Ankle Mobs

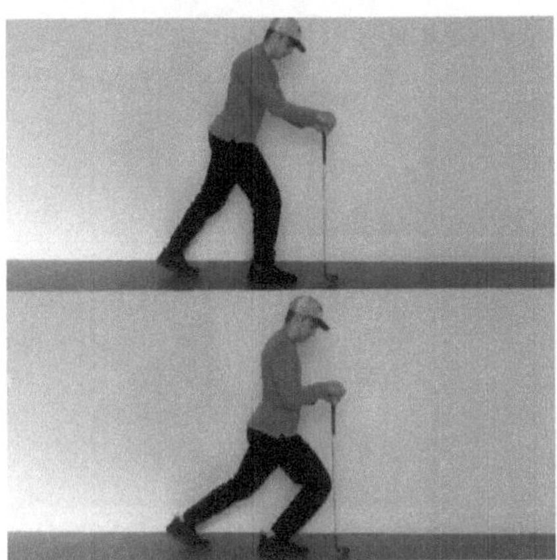

To Perform...

-Place the front of the foot about 6 inches away from the golf club or wall if available

-Keeping the lead foot flat, try and touch the knee to the golf club or wall

Lateral - Leg Swings

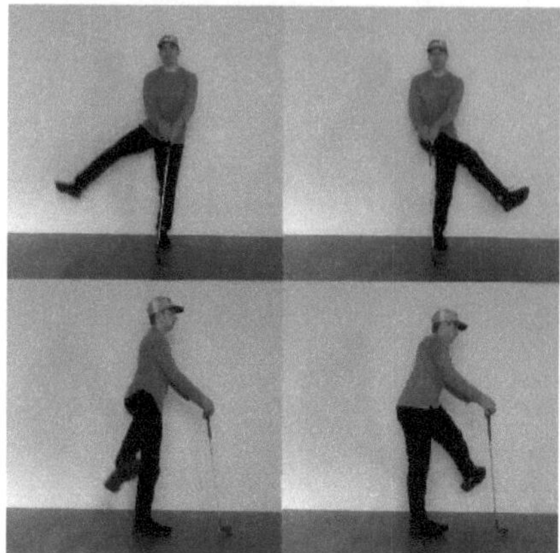

To Perform…

-Place the hands on the golf club or against the wall and swing one leg side to side

-Make sure the leg on the ground stays straight

Knee (Stable Joint):

Phase 1: Supine Knee Flexion/Extension

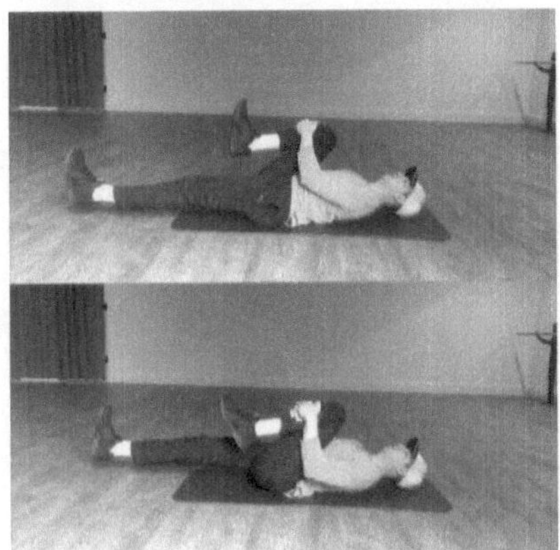

To Perform...

-Hug one leg and bring it towards the chest

-Extend the opposite leg (Should be 1 inch off the ground)

Phase 2: Quadruped Single Leg Extension

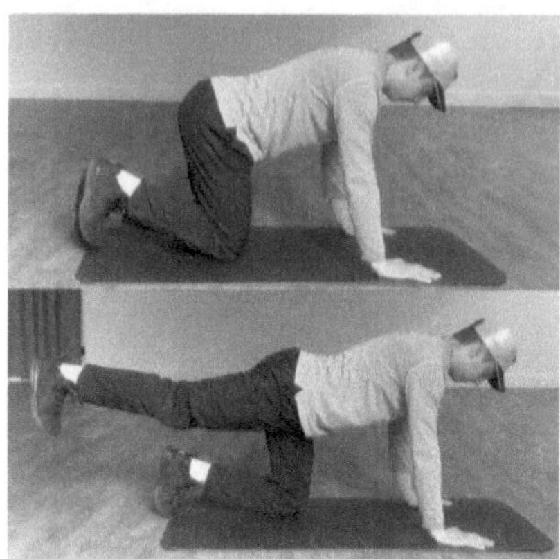

To Perform...

-Start from the quadruped position (hands directly below shoulders and knees directly below shoulders)

-Extend one leg directly backwards so that it is parallel with the floor (**Feel like the leg is pushing a box away from the body**)

Phase 3:

Standing Quad Pull w/Straight Leg + Standing Single Leg Hip Flexion

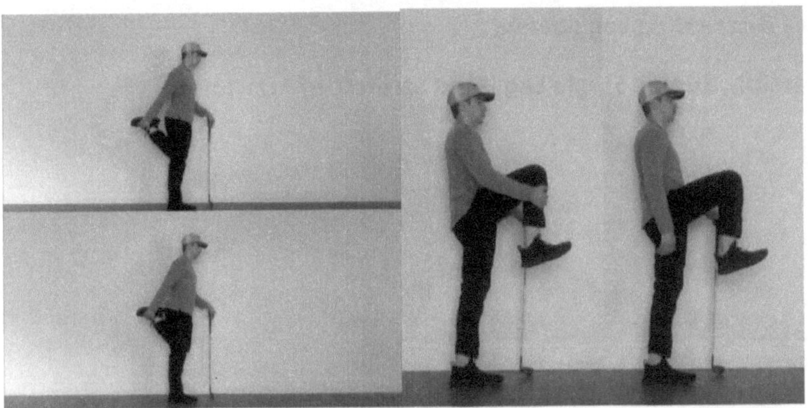

To Perform...

Standing Quad Pull w/Straight Leg (Left)

-Use the golf club to support and help balance

-Pull one leg towards the butt and hold

-Keep the leg straight that is on the ground

Standing Single Leg Hip Flexion (Right)

-Use the golf club to support and help balance

-Pull one leg towards the chest while keeping the leg straight

-Let go of the leg and try to actively keep it at the same height

Hip (Mobile Joint):

Phase 1:

Linear - Alternating Leg Lowers

(Regression: Supine Single Leg Band Stretch w/Activation)

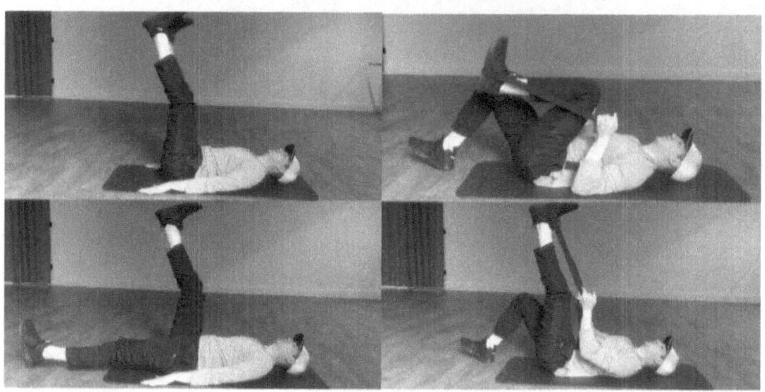

To Perform...

Leg Lower (Left)

-Raise the legs up to the sky and keep them as straight as possible

-Push the hands into the ground and lower one leg

-Raise the leg back up and then proceed to alternate each repetition

Supine Single Leg Band Stretch w/Hamstring Activation (Right)

-Place the band or strap around the middle of the foot

-Pull knee towards the chest

-Then push into the band and straighten the leg

Lateral – Supine Hip Circles or Passive Straight Leg Twist

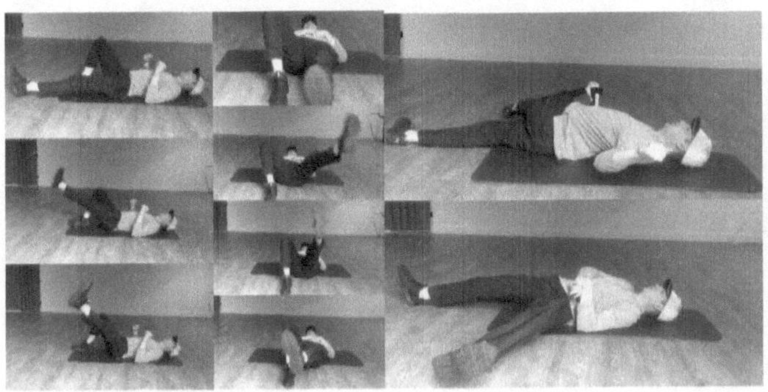

To Perform...

Supine Hip Circles (Left)

-Place one foot flat on the ground and extend the opposing leg

-Keeping the leg straight, circle the leg both ways

Passive Straight Leg Twist (Right)

-Place the band around the center of foot

-Keep the leg straight and rotate the hip to the left and then to the right

Phase 2:

Linear – Quadruped Hip Extension

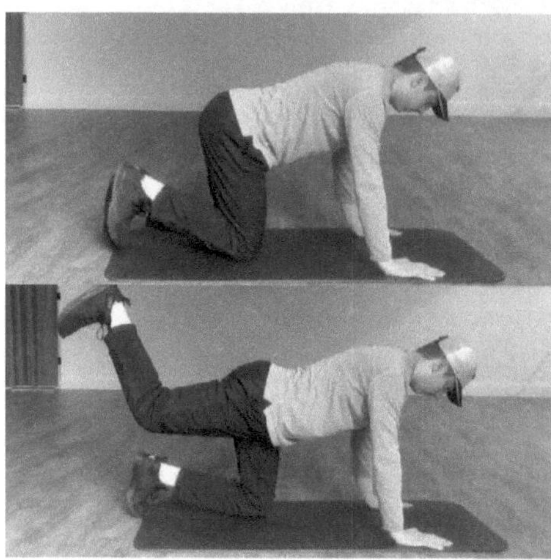

To Perform...

-Place the hands directly below the shoulders and knees directly below the hips

-Try to keep a 90-degree angle between the hamstring (back of the upper half of the leg) and calf (back of the lower half of the leg)

-Extend the heel up towards the sky

Lateral – Quadruped Hip Circles

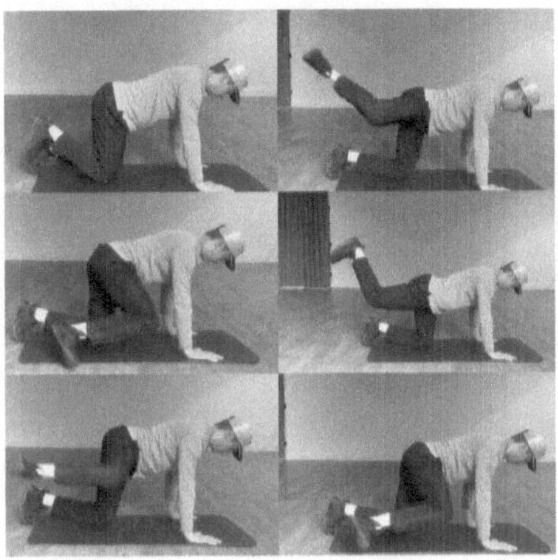

To Perform…

-From the quadruped position bring the moving knee towards the lead elbow

-Trace the knee in a circular motion and then reverse it back to the starting position

-Feel like there is a hurdle to the side of the leg and that the knee is going up and over it

Phase 3:

Linear - Toe Touches (Full Extension)

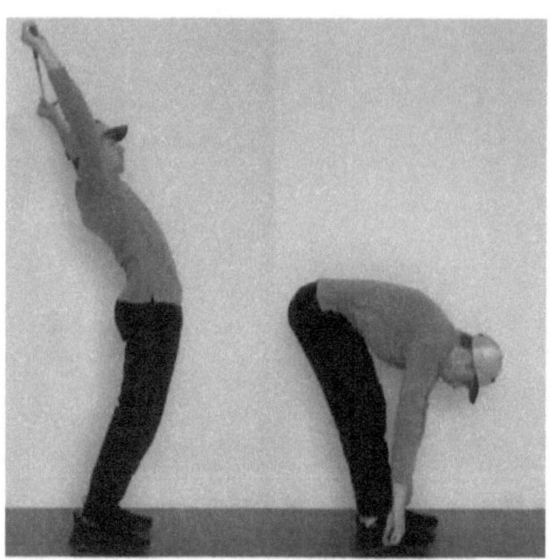

To Perform...

-Place hands on the golf club a little wider than shoulder width

-Extend the hips forward and reach the hands backwards

-Then reverse the motion and proceed to touch the toes

Lateral – Standing Hip Circles or Stork Turns

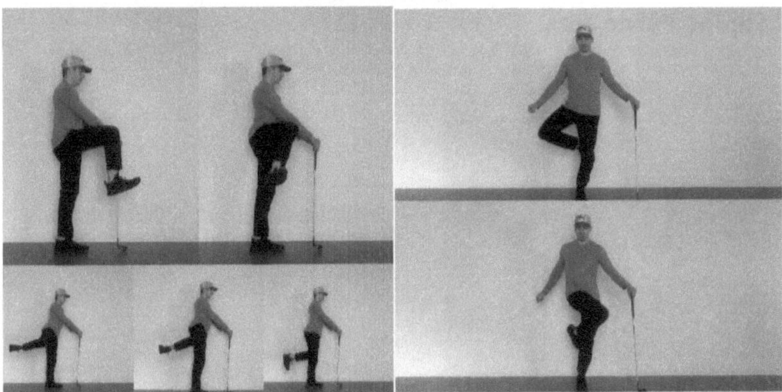

To Perform...

Hip Circles (Left)

-Place hands on golf club or wall for support

-Bring the knee directly upward

-Then open the hip up while keeping the chest facing forward

-From there keep tracing a circle with the knee and reverse it from the bottom position

Stork Turns (Right)

-Use the golf club or wall for support

-Place one foot behind the knee and rotate the hip side to side while keeping the chest facing forward

Lower Back (Stable Joint):

Phase 1: Supine Pelvic Tilts

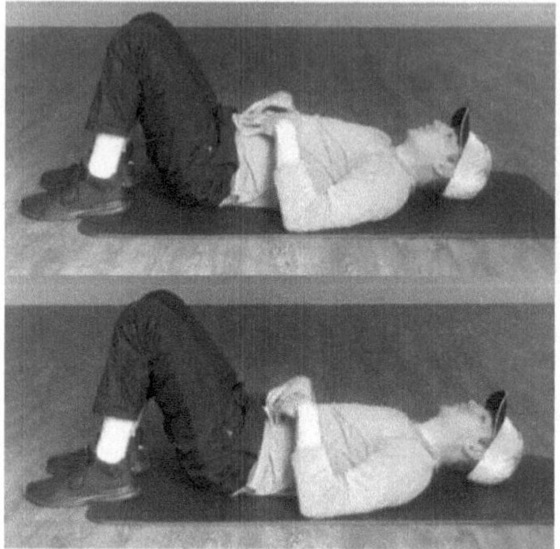

To Perform...

-Breathe in and expand the stomach to the sky

-Breathe out and tuck the stomach into the floor

Phase 2: Cat & Camels

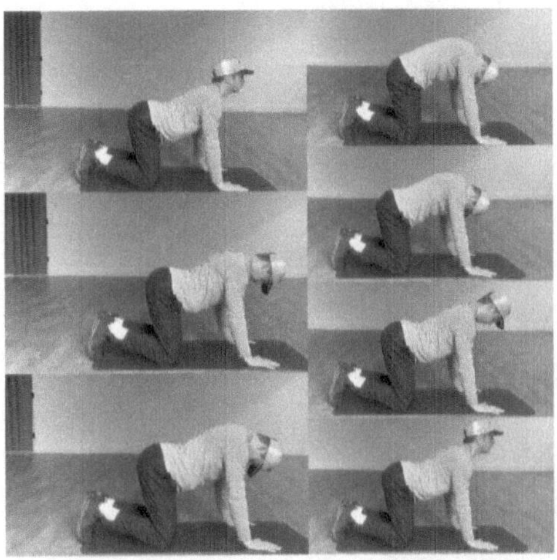

To Perform...

-From the quadruped position sink the spine towards the ground and neck up towards the sky

-Start by tilting the neck downward and then slowly inch the spine upward from there

-At the top, the neck is tilted down, and the upper and lower spine form an arch that is reaching toward the sky

-Then proceed to start the downward position by tilting down from the lowest part of the spine

-From there slowly inch on upward from the spine until the spine ends up in the starting position

Phase 3: Standing Pelvic Tilts

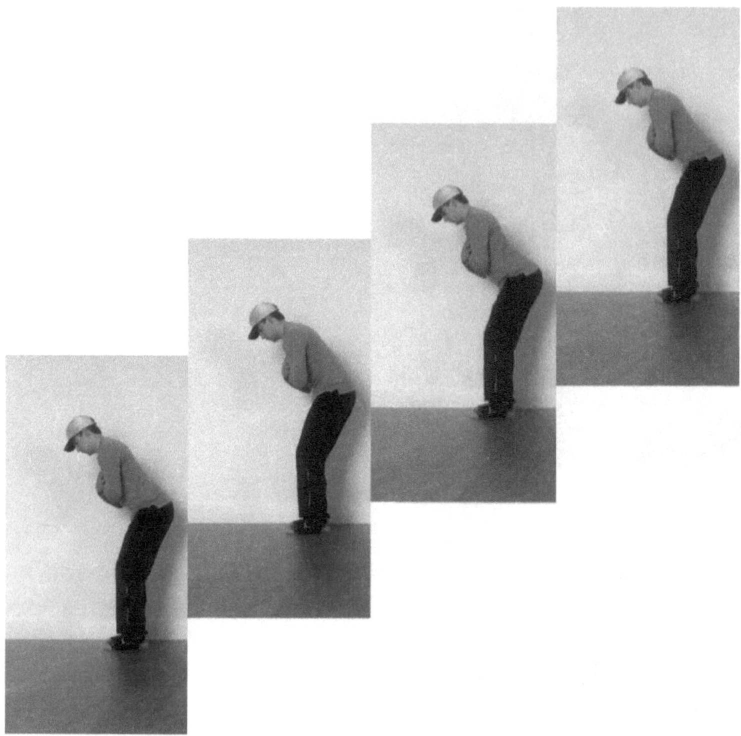

To Perform…

-Place the hands across the chest in golf posture

-Start with a neutral spine and tilt the stomach away from the ground

-From there, reverse the tilt so that the spine is arched, and the belly button is pointed toward the ground

-Find neutral and then repeat

T-Spine (Mobile Joint):

Phase 1:

Supine Arm Bar (Progression: Add Kettlebell)

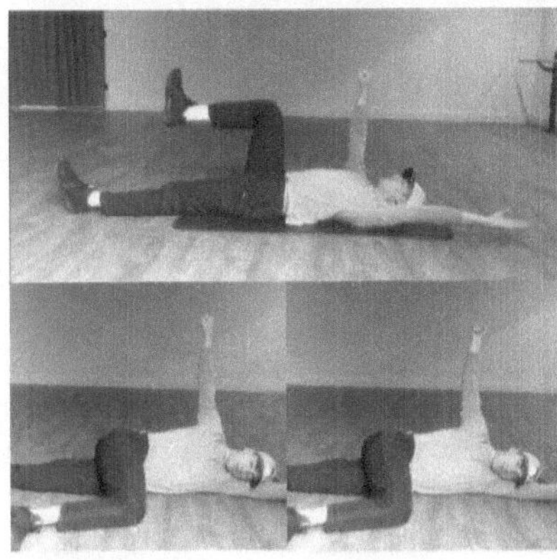 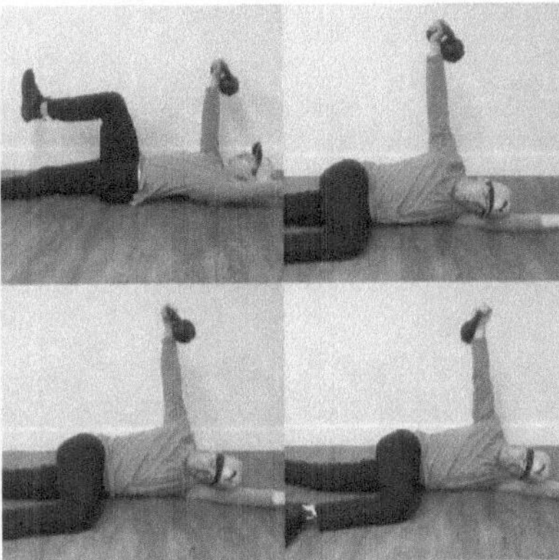

To Perform…

-Place one leg at a 90-degree angle and place the hand on the same side in the air

-Slowly allow the leg in the air to rotate towards the opposing side

-Once settled, proceed to rotate the shoulder inward and outward

Regression: For Supine Arm Bar

Side-Lying Open Books + Supine Protractions and Retractions

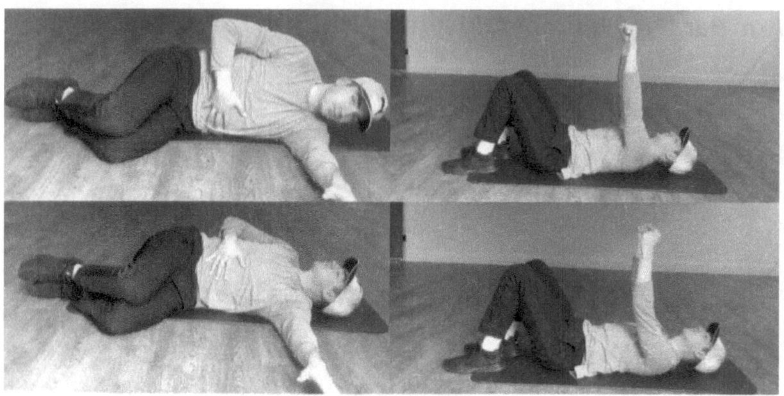

To Perform...

Side-Lying Open Books (Left)

-Lay on the side and place the hand of the raised shoulder on the stomach

-With the knee and hand that are touching the ground proceed to press them into the ground with about 70% pressure

-Then open the chest and shoulder toward the ground

-Allow the neck to open as well

Supine Protractions and Retractions (Right)

-Simply reach the hands up to the sky

-Then twist the hands inward and bring them towards the ground

Phase 2:

Quadruped T-Spine External Rotation

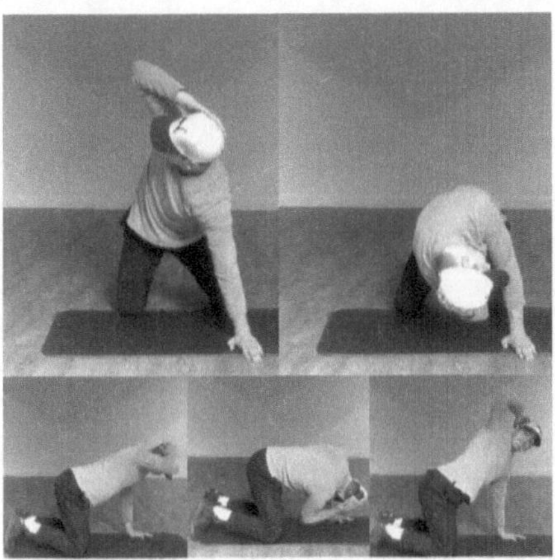

To Perform...

-From the quadruped position place one hand behind the head

-Reach that elbow downward towards the opposite knee

-Then proceed to reach the moving elbow up toward the sky

-Important that the eyes follow the elbow that is moving the entire time

Optional Progression: Half-Kneeling T-Spine Rotations

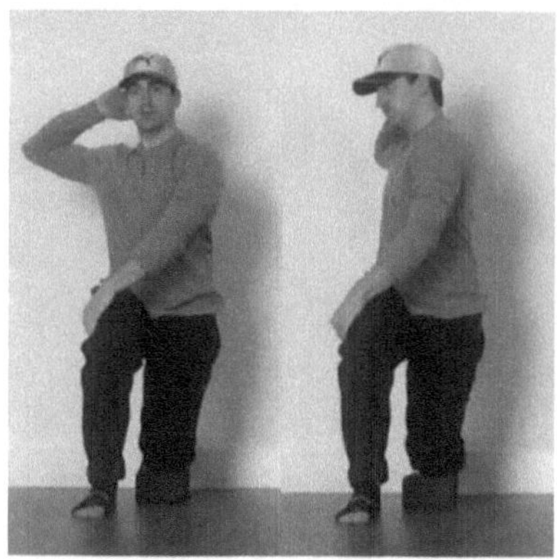

To Perform...

-From the half-kneeling position, place the opposite hand on the lead knee

-Place the other hand behind the head

-Staying as upright as possible, proceed to twist as far as possible

Phase 3:

A-Frame Stretch or Bent Over T-Spine External Rotations

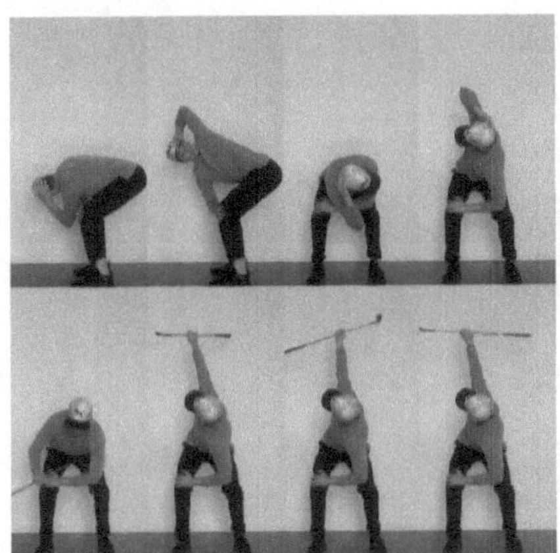

To Perform...

T-Spine External Rotations (Top)

-Place the elbow and hand on the knees and the opposite hand behind the head

-Keeping the lower body still, rotate the upper body downward and then reverse it back upward

A-Frame Stretch (Bottom)

- Place the elbow and hand on the knees and the opposite hand reaching towards the sky with a golf club

-Rotate the golf club back and forth, mostly by using the shoulder

Scapula (Stable Joint):

Phase 1:

Supine Floor Slides + Supine Arm Reaches

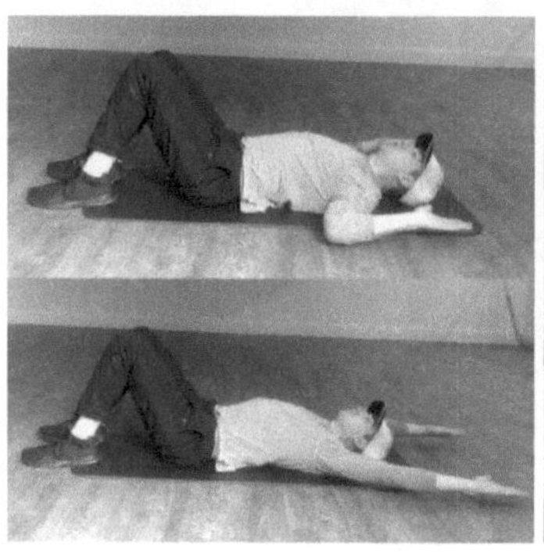 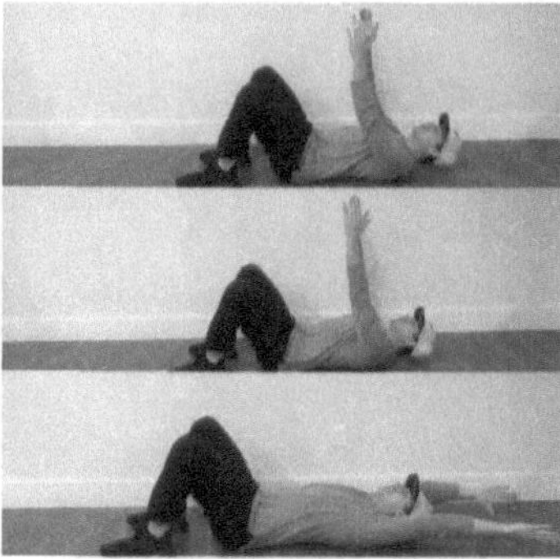

To Perform...

Supine Floor Slides (Left)

-Push the feet into the floor and press the elbows and wrist against the ground

-Take a deep breath in

-Straighten the arms as you breathe out

Supine Arm Reaches (Right)

-Point the thumbs away from the body

-Reach the arms up towards the sky

-Keep reaching the arms away from the body as they raise overhead

Phase 2:

Half-Kneeling Single Arm Reach + Half-Kneeling Elevation and Depression

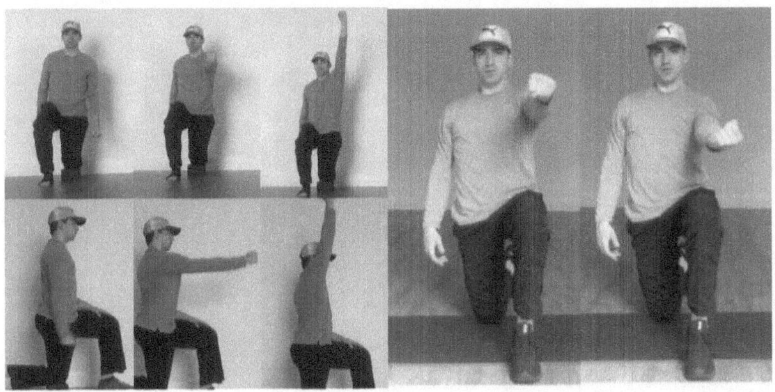

To Perform...

Half-Kneeling Single Arm Reach (Left)

-From the half-kneeling position make a fist with the hand opposite of the lead foot

-Keep the moving arm straight and reach it forward, then on upward

Half-Kneeling Elevation and Depression (Right)

-From the half-kneeling position make a fist with the same hand as the lead foot

-Twist the arm downward (shaping a C) while keeping the arm straight

-This movement should come mostly from the shoulder

Phase 3:

Standing Wall Slides or Arm Raise w/Golf Club + Standing Arm Reaches

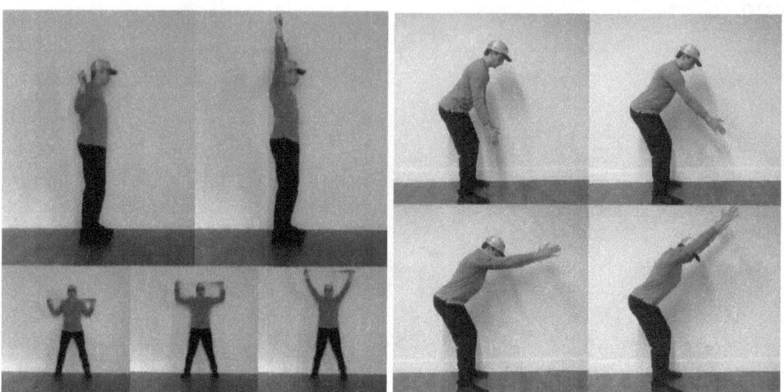

To Perform…

Standing Wall Slides (Left)

-Grip the club a little wider than shoulder width and place it behind the head

-Take a deep breath and tuck the stomach inward

-Breathe out and extend the club towards the sky

Standing Arm Reaches (Right)

-Reach the hands toward the ground and away from the body

-Slowly raise the arms up to an overhead position

-Keep the arms straight the entire time

Shoulder (Mobile Joint):

Phase 1: *Supine Arm Bar w/Internal and External Rotation (Progression: Add Kettlebell)

-This movement is targeted in a two-in-one exercise listed above which is the "Supine Arm Bar w/Internal and External Rotation"

Phase 2: Half-Kneeling Arm Circle

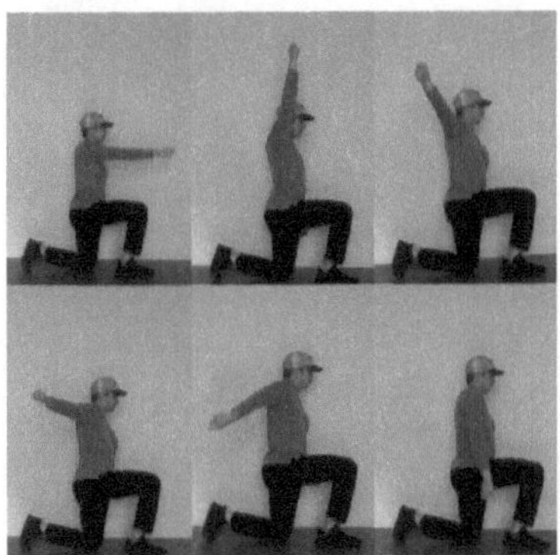

To Perform...

-From the half-kneeling position reach the arm directly in front of the body and as far forward as possible

-Pretend there is a pencil in the hand and draw the biggest circle possible

-At the top position rotate the hand away from the body

-At the bottom position reverse the circle

Phase 3: Tom House Arm Circle Circuit

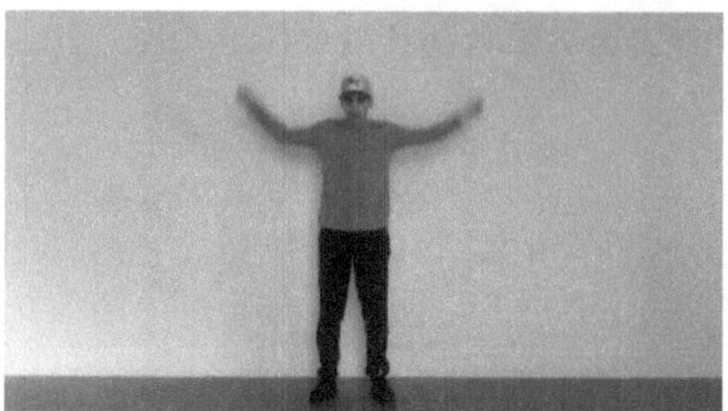

To Perform...

-Slightly bend the elbows and circle the arms

-There are small, medium, and large arms circles performed both forward and backwards for the prescribed amount of time

Wrist (Mobile Joint)/Elbow (Stable Joint):

Phase 1:

Supine Wrist Press Ups

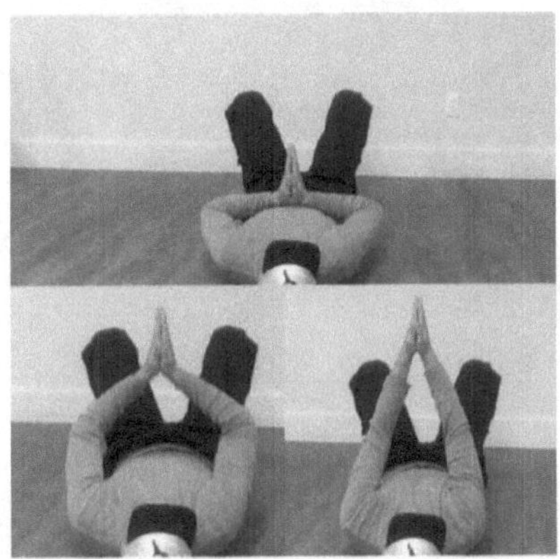

To Perform...

Supine Wrist Press Ups

-Press the palm of the hands together while keeping the forearms parallel to the ground

-Apply about 70% pressure to the hands and straighten the arms to the sky

Ulnar and Radial Wrist Flexion + Supine Wrist Flexion and Extension

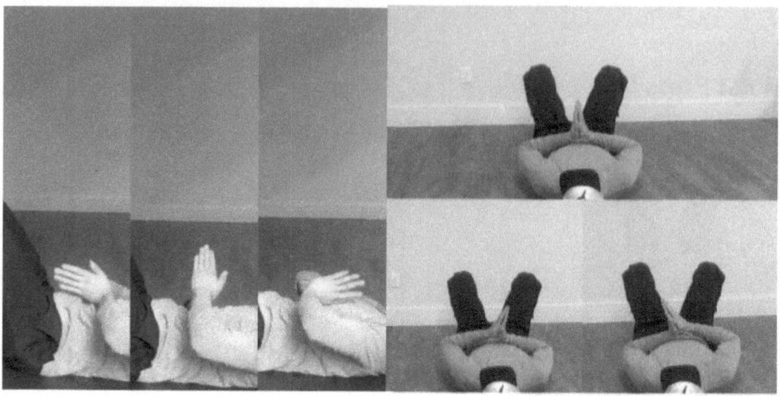

To Perform...

Ulnar and Radial Wrist Flexion (Left)

-Press the palm of the hands together and rotate the hands towards the chin and then back towards the feet

Supine Wrist Flexion and Extension (Right)

-Press the palm of the hands together while keeping the forearms as close to parallel to the ground as possible

-Flex and extend the wrist to the right and left

Phase 2:

Quadruped Wrist Mobs (Flexion & Extension)

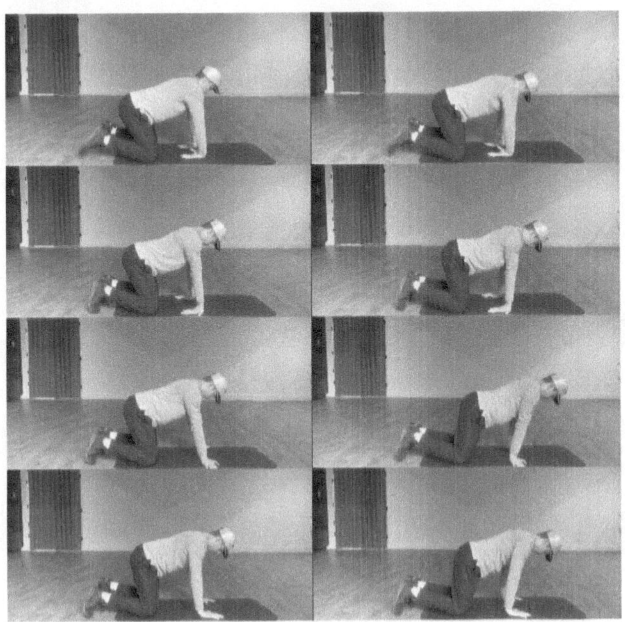

To Perform...

-From the quadruped position rock back and forth with the...

*Knuckles to the ground (Top Photos)

*Palms to the ground facing the knees (Top-Middle Photos)

*Palms to the ground with hands facing outward (Bottom-Middle Photos)

*Palms to the ground with hands pointing away from the body (Bottom Photos)

Phase 3:

Elbow/Wrist - Power Three 3 w/Golf Club

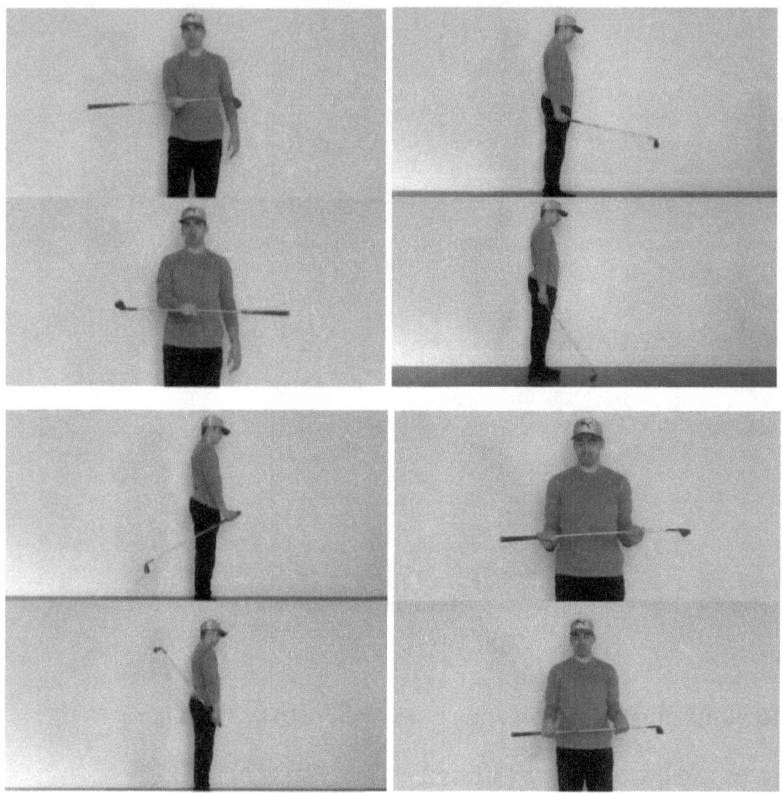

To Perform...

Pronation and Supination (Top Left)

-Place the elbow on the side of the body

-Rotate the hand inward and outward

Ulnar Deviation (Top Right)

-With the club in front of the body, flex the wrist towards the sky and then extend downward

Radial Deviation (Bottom Left)

-With the club behind the body, flex the wrist towards the sky and then extend downward

Wrist Extension and Flexion (Bottom Right)

-Grip the club with the hands about shoulder width apart and extend them upward and then flex downward

Neck (Mobile Joint)

Phase 1:

Linear – Supine Neck Flexion and Extension

Lateral – Supine Side to Side Neck Rotations

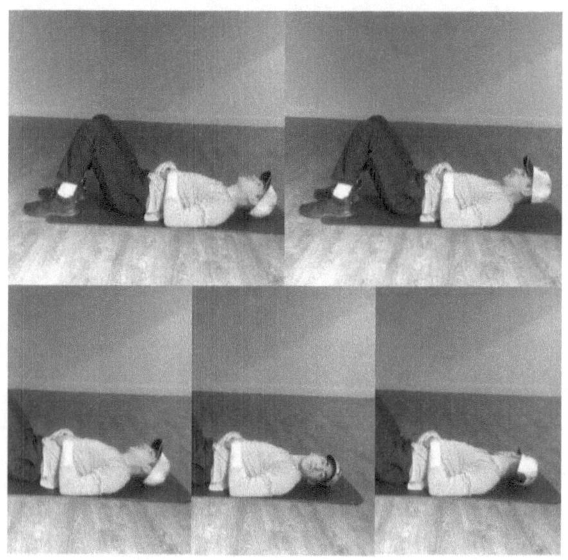

Supine Neck Flexion and Extension (Top)

-Slightly tuck chin upward (*not all the way)

Supine Side to Side Neck Rotations (Bottom)

-Simply twist the neck to the left and right

Phase 2:

Linear – Quadruped Flexion and Extension (*Cat & Camel)

-This movement is targeted in a two-in-one exercise listed above which is the "Cat & Camel"

Lateral – Quadruped Side to Side w/Chin to Sternum or Tall-Kneeling Side to Side Twist w/Chin to Sternum

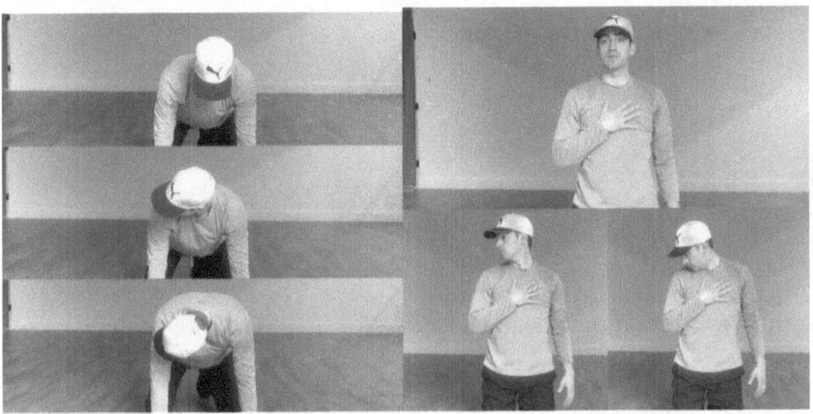

To Perform...

Quadruped Side to Side Neck Twist

-From the quadruped position rotate the neck toward one shoulder

-Then proceed to tuck the chin towards the clavicle

Tall-Kneeling Side to Side Twist w/Chin to Sternum

-In the tall-kneeling position twist the neck toward the opposite shoulder

-Tilt the chin toward the clavicle

Phase 3:

Linear + Lateral - Standing Neck Circles

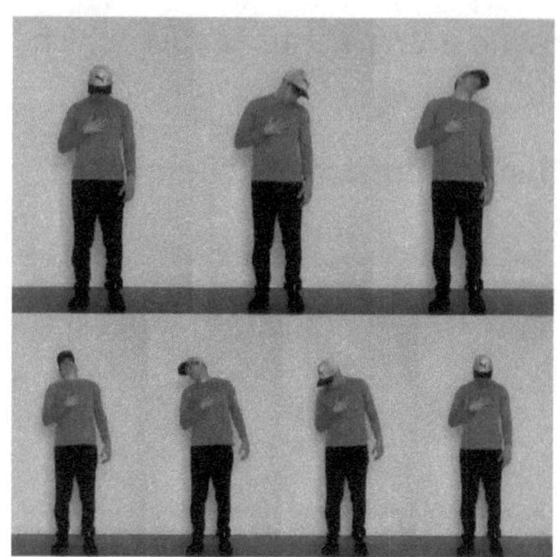

To Perform...

-Close the mouth and place the shoulders back behind the body (Standing Tall Position)

-Make a slow circle with the neck then switch direction

Movement Circuit:

Once the mobility is primed, it's important to ensure that the tissue temperature of the muscles are increased to allow them to absorb and adapt to stress better, but also to make sure the body is mentally prepared through appropriate activation of the central nervous system (CNS). As stated above the CNS consist of the brain and spinal cord and helps coordinate the body to execute the movements it would like to perform.

The movement circuit consists of both linear (straight) and lateral (side to side) movement patterns to ensure that multiple planes of motion are targeted throughout the program.

The circuit breakdown will include the following exercises….

1.) A **lower** or **upper body power** exercise
2.) A **core** stability exercise
3.) A **lower body** stability exercise
4.) A **coordination** exercise

LOWER POWER

Phase 1:

Jump Squats

(Regression – Perform everything the same just don't jump)

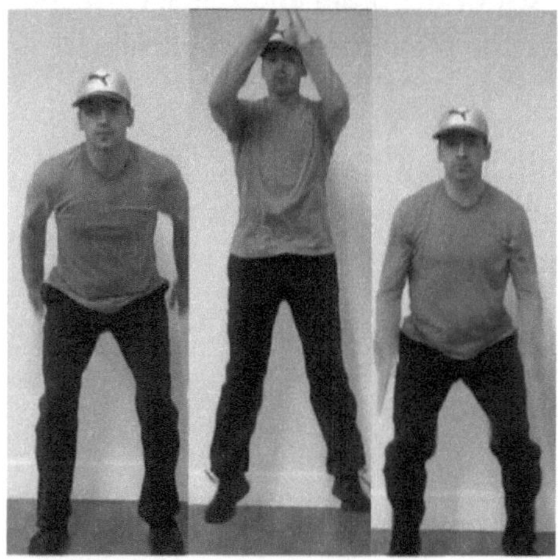

To Perform:

-Load the lower body by bringing the hands back and shifting the weight towards the heels of the feet

-Then explode up and move the hands upward for increased momentum

Phase 2:

Single Leg Jump Squat w/Bilateral Landing

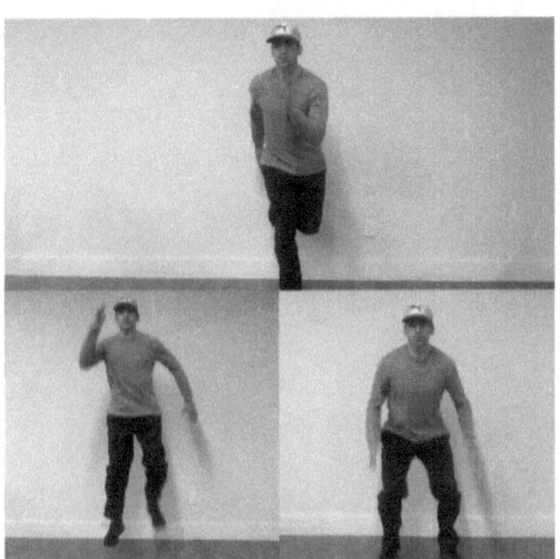

To Perform:

-Stand on one leg

-With the leg that is on the ground place the same side hand behind the body

-Jump up and use the hands to create momentum

-Land on two feet

Phase 3:

Single Leg Jump Squats

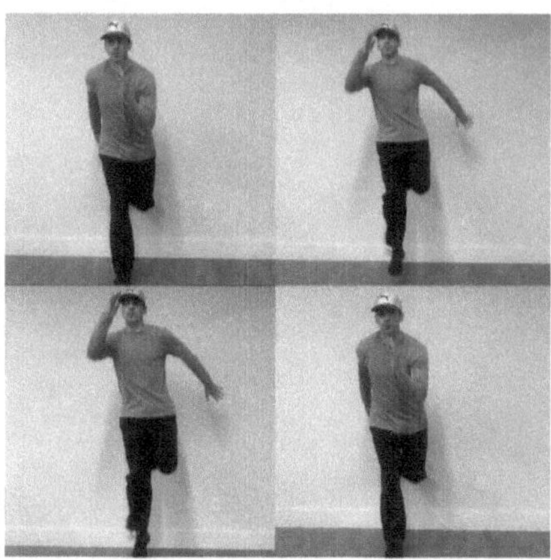

To Perform...

-Stand on one leg

-With the leg that is on the ground place the same side hand behind the body

-Jump up and use the hands to create momentum

-Land on one foot and place the hands right back where they started

LINEAR CORE

Phase 1:

Push-Up Hold

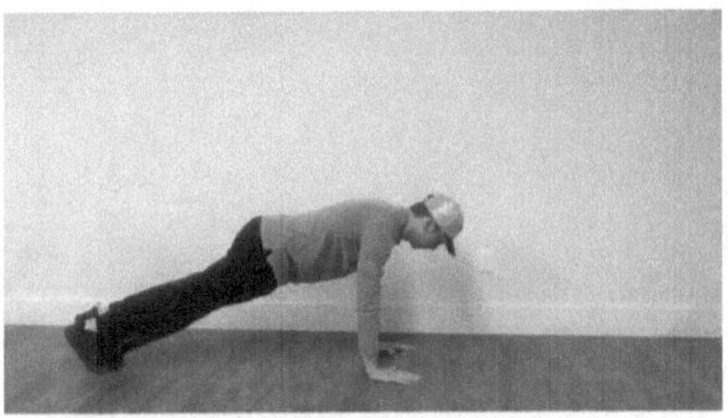

To Perform...

-Get into the push-up position with the hands directly over the shoulders

-Breathe in through the nose and fill the upper back with air

-Then breathe out through the mouth and feel like the hands are twisting outward away from the body.

Phase 2:

Plank

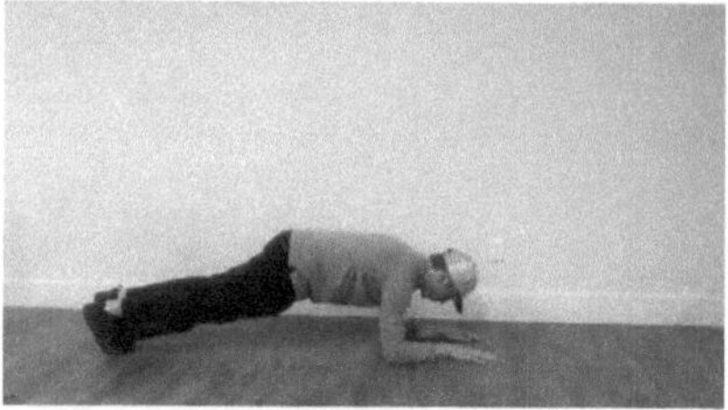

To Perform...

-Place the elbows directly below the shoulders while pressing the toes into the ground

-Breathe in through the nose and fill the upper back with air

-Then breathe out through the mouth and feel like the elbows are sliding towards the feet

Phase 3:

Long Lever Plank

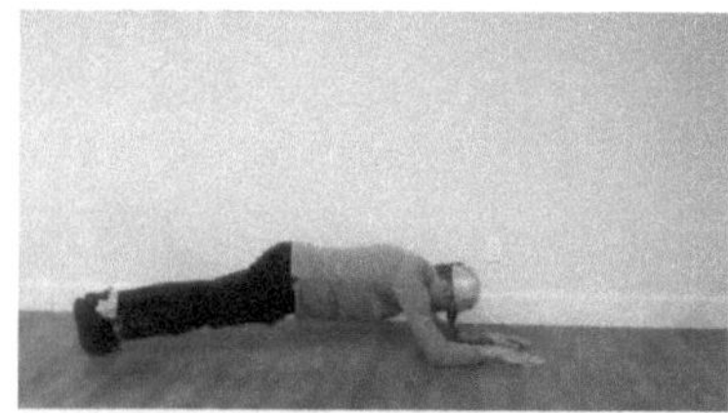

To Perform...

-Place the elbows slightly in front (higher) of the shoulders

-Breathe in through the nose and out through the mouth

LINEAR LOWER

Phase 1:

Single Leg Cook Hip Lift

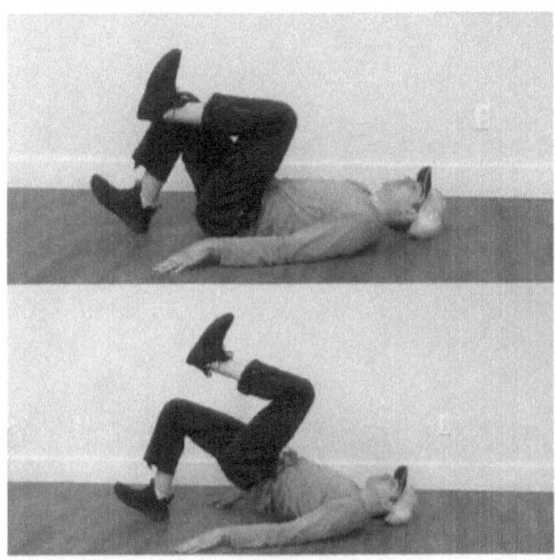

To Perform...

-Lying on the back, dig one heel into the ground while pulling the other knee toward the chest.

-Push the hands into the ground and slightly away from the body

-Then lift the hips up

Phase 2:

Single Leg Cook Hip Lift Holds

To Perform...

-Repeat same steps as the single leg cook hip lift except hold it for the prescribed amount of time

Phase 3:

Single Leg Bucks

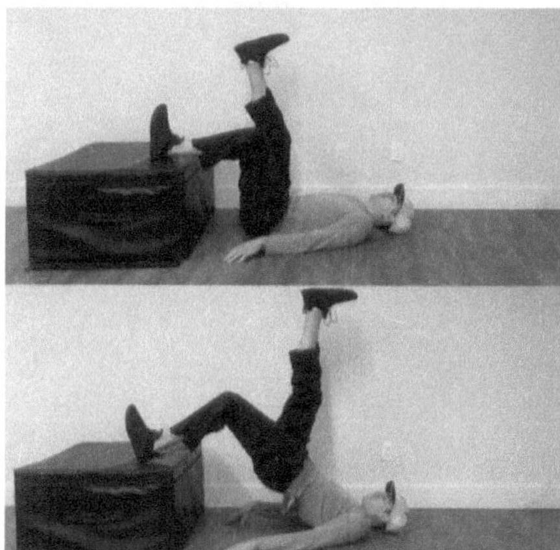

To Perform...

-Use a box, bench, or something sturdy to support the leg at a 90-degree angle

-Then press the hands into the ground and the heel in to the box

-Proceed to lift the hip off the ground

LINEAR COORDINTION

Phase 1:

Bird Dogs

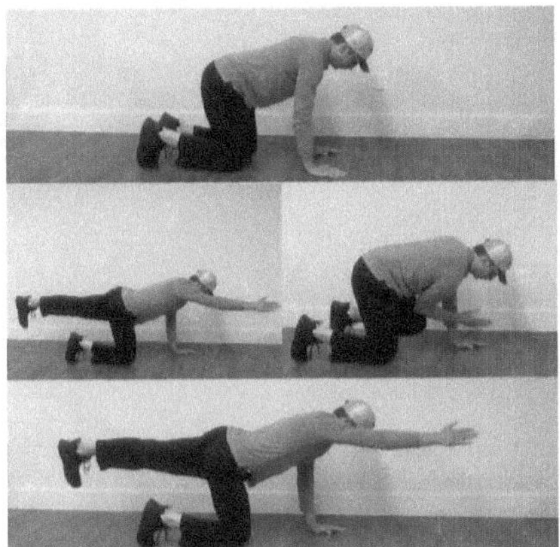

To Perform...

-Get into the quadruped position

-Reach the opposite arm and leg out, staying as steady as possible

-Then touch the elbow to knee and repeat the same side for the prescribed amount of reps before switching sides

Phase 2:

Bird Dog Holds

To Perform...

-Repeat the same steps as the bird dogs but hold the extended arm and leg position for the prescribed amount of reps

Phase 3:

Bird Dog w/No Feet

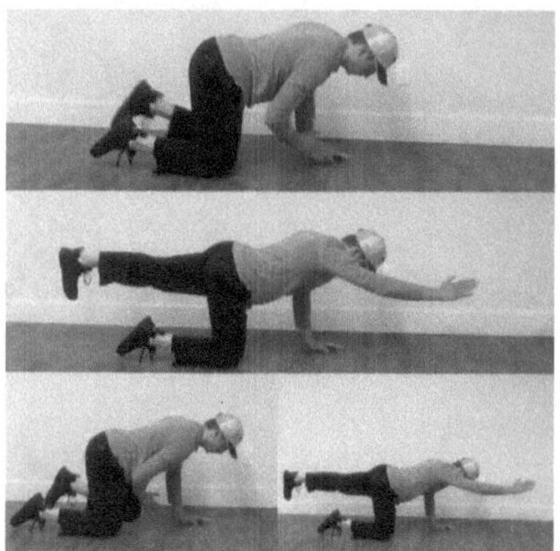

To Perform...

-Repeat the same steps as the bird dog except lift the toes off the ground

-Also, when coming inward touch the hand to the knee instead of the elbow to the knee

UPPER POWER

Phase 1:

Half-Kneeling Rotational Throw w/Band

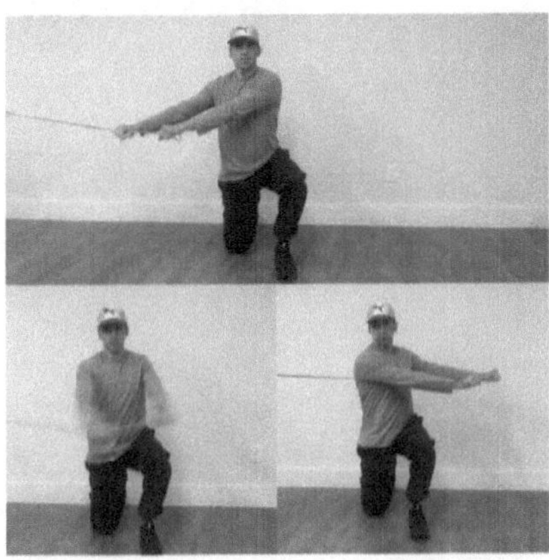

To Perform...

-Place the band about chest height and attach it to something sturdy

-From there get into the half-kneeling position

-Grip the band about shoulder width apart, with the palms facing the ground (motorcycle grip)

-Then proceed to rotate the upper body and bring the band past the lead leg as fast as possible

-Pause at the finish position and slowly bring the band back to the starting position

Phase 2:

Standing Rotational Throw w/Band

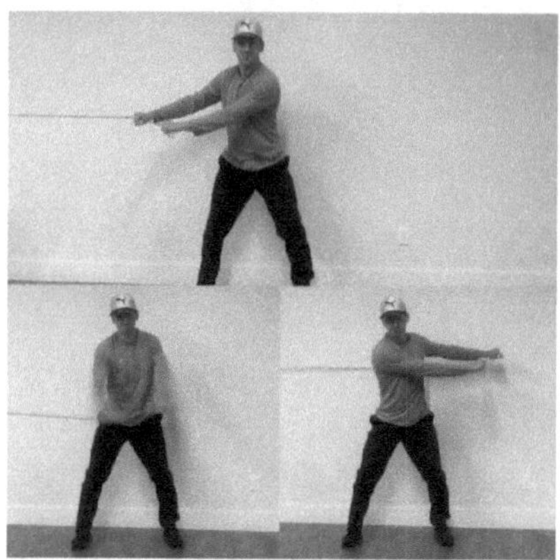

To Perform…

-Repeat the same steps as the half-kneeling throw w/band, except from the standing position

-Also, keep the lower body fairly still

Phase 3:

Stepping Rotational Throw w/Band

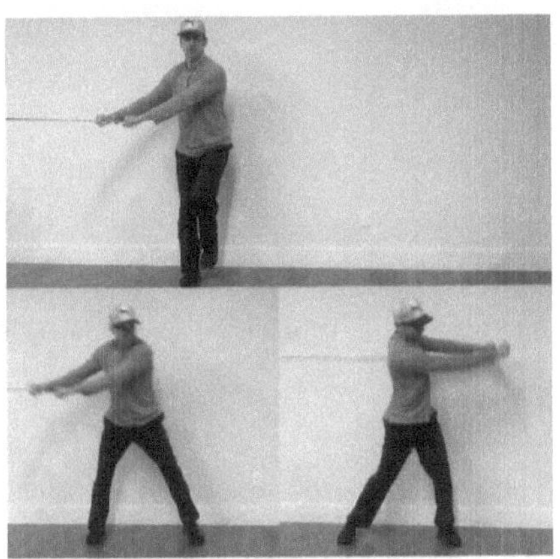

To Perform...

-Repeat the same steps as the half-kneeling throw w/band except with the lead foot stepping forward

-Also, the lower body should rotate with this exercise

LATERAL CORE

Phase 1:

Side Plank from Knees

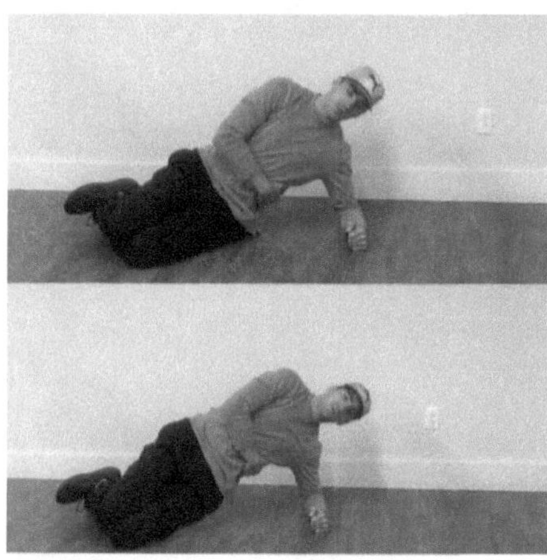

To Perform...

-Place the knees in front of the chest and the feet behind the hips

-Then place the top hand on the bottom external obliques (side of the abdomen)

-Once the following are in place, proceed to push the forearm, knee, and outside of foot into the ground

-Then lift the hip up in to the position in the picture above

Phase 2:

Side Plank from Knees w/Abduction

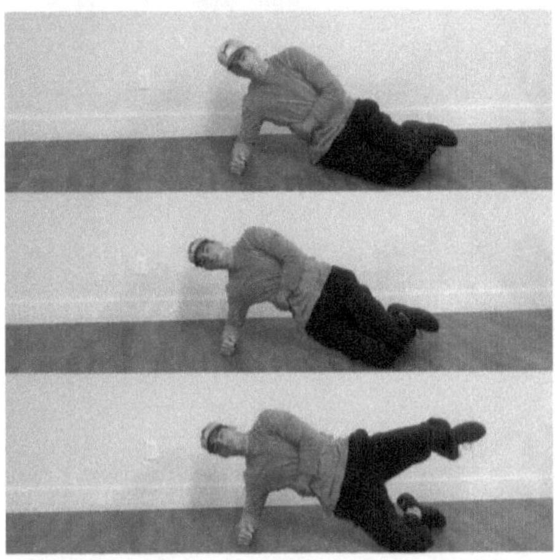

To Perform...

-Perform the same steps as the side plank from knees except lift the top knee and foot up

Phase 3:

Side Plank

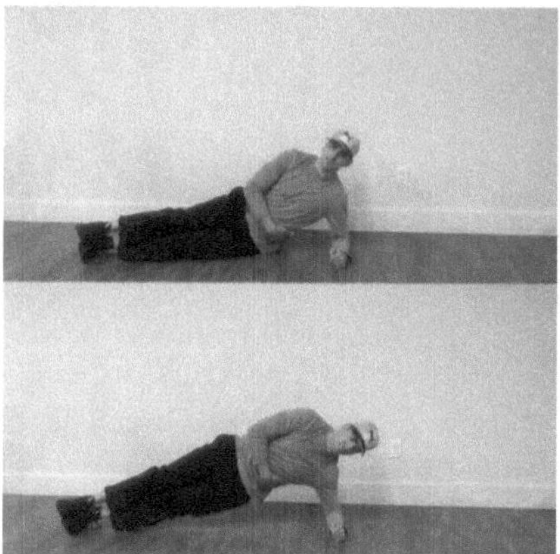

To Perform...

-Place the elbow below the shoulder and stack the feet on each other

-Then place the top hand on the bottom external oblique (side of the abdomen)

-Press the forearm and the outside of the foot into the floor

-Then proceed to lift the hip up

LATERAL LOWER

Phase 1:

Assisted Lateral Lunge

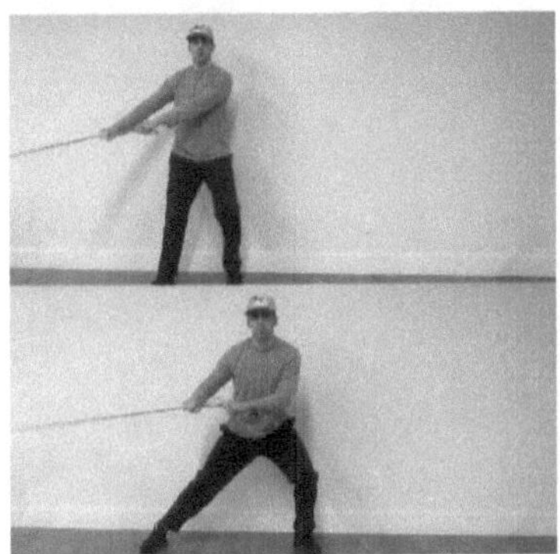

-Place the band about chest to hip height on something sturdy

-Hold the band in a comfortable position and step out to the side

-Straighten the trail leg and sink into the hip of the leg that is stepping out

-Make sure the weight is mostly towards the heel of the foot stepping out but also that the knee is directly above the ankle at the bottom position

Phase 2:

Lateral Lunge w/Step

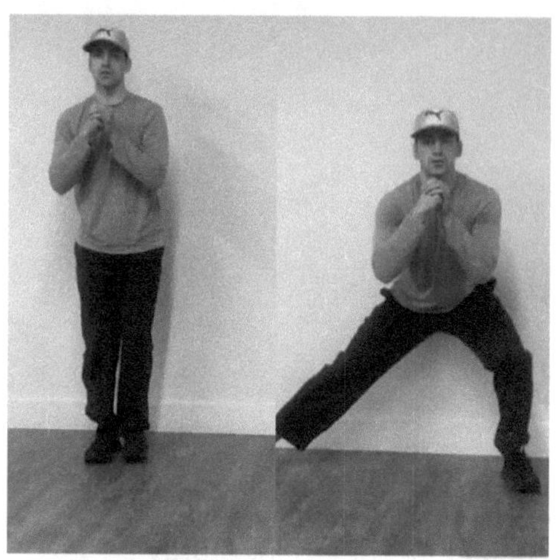

To Perform…

-Repeat the steps from the assisted lateral lunge except without the band

Phase 3:

Lateral Lunge w/Band Pressout

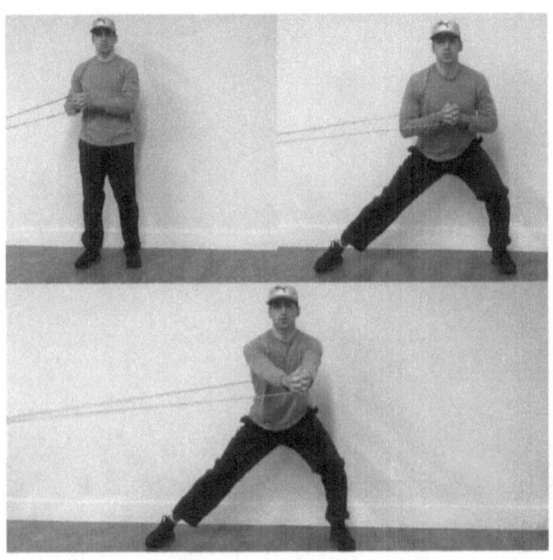

To Perform...

-Repeat the steps from the assisted lateral lunge except at the bottom position press the hand and band straight out

LATERAL COORDINATION

Phase 1:

Single Leg Balance

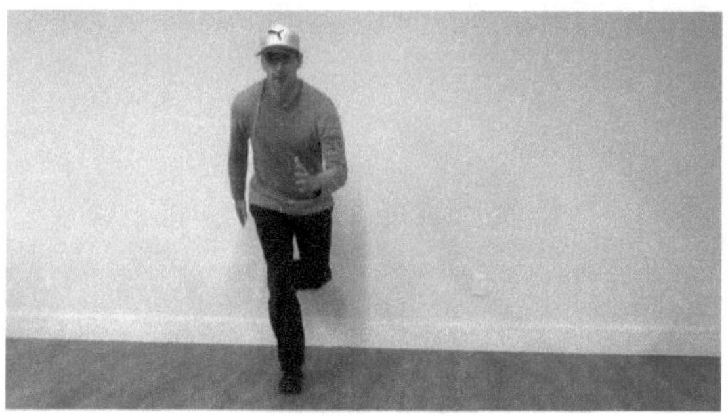

To Perform…

-While balancing on one leg, make sure the foot, knee, and hip are directly over each other

-Then place the same hand as the foot on the ground behind the hips and the other hand forward

Phase 2:

Single Leg Balance w/Alternating Reach

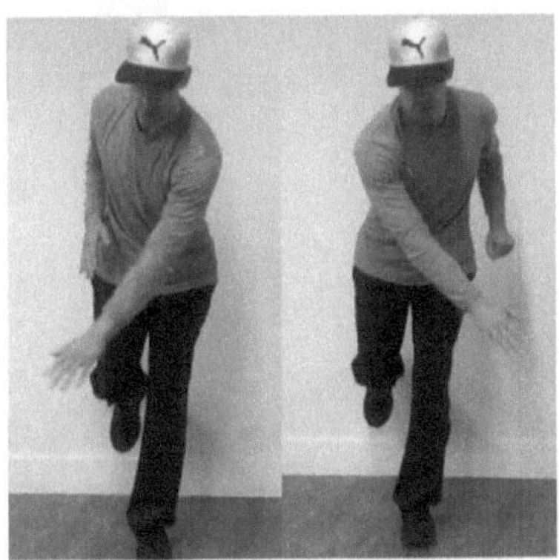

To Perform...

-Repeat the steps from the single leg balance except alternate reaching left and right

Phase 3:

Single Leg Balance w/Rotation

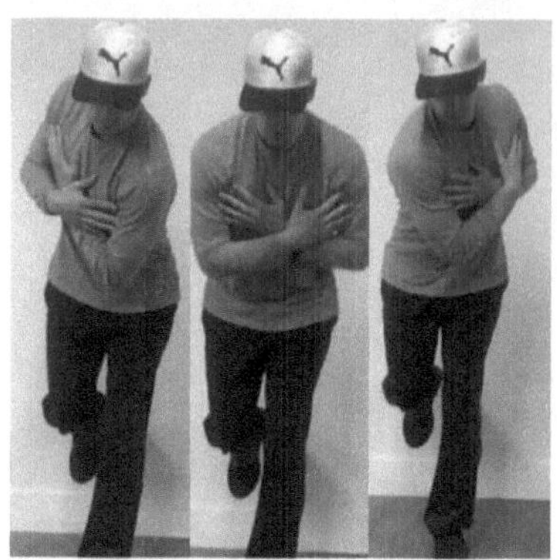

To Perform...

-Repeat the steps from the single leg balance except place the hands across the chest and rotate the upper body while keeping the lower body as still as possible

Chapter 5: Progressive Strength Training Program

Strength training made simple would be:

Safely progress an overload on the muscles = Increased Strength

That's it, overload the muscles in a safe manner and you will be forced to get stronger. With a progressive system like the one listed below, the body will be able to adapt and get stronger.

The exercises are designed to target the entire body through pushing and pulling patterns with the lower and upper body. There are also accessory exercises to make sure the core and smaller muscles--like the calf and rotator cuff--get targeted.

The exercise categories include:

<u>Upper Body</u>

Vertical Push Movements: Ex.) Single Arm Band Overhead Press

Horizontal Push Movements: Ex.) Single Arm Band Press

Vertical Pull Movements: Ex.) Half-Kneeling Band Pulldown

Horizontal Pull Movements: Ex.) Half-Kneeling Band Row

<u>Lower Body</u>

Single Leg Knee Dominant (**Squat**) – Split Squat

Bilateral Knee Dominant (**Squat**) – Band Overhead Squat

Single Leg Hip Dominant (**Hip Hinge**) – Single Leg Deadlift

Bilateral Hip Dominant (**Hip Hinge**) – Band Romanian Deadlift

<u>Core</u>

Anti-Lateral Flexion: Ex.) Half-Kneeling Anti-Lateral Flexion Hold

Anti-Rotation: Ex.) Half-Kneeling Anti-Rotation Press

Chop/Lift: Ex.) Half-Kneeling Chop

82

<u>Accessory</u>

Calves/Tib Anterior – Ex.) Single Leg Calf Raise

Rotator Cuff – Ex.) Single Arm Band Pullapart

Together these movements will target all three planes of motion that the body can move in. These planes of motion include the sagittal (direct movement forward or backward), frontal (direct movement left or right), and transverse (rotational movement).

Sagittal Plane Movement

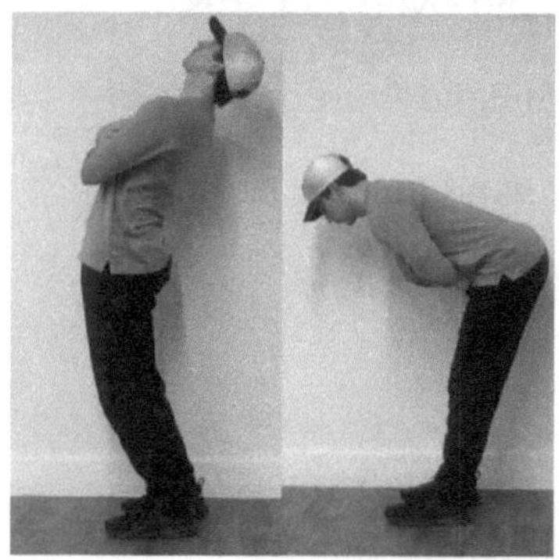

Frontal Plane Movement

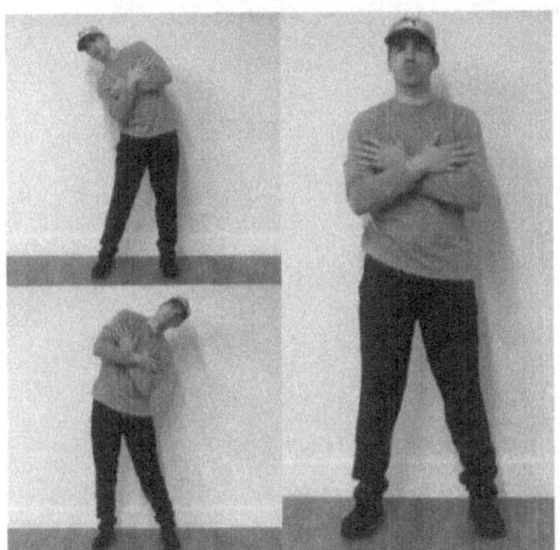

Transverse Plane Movement

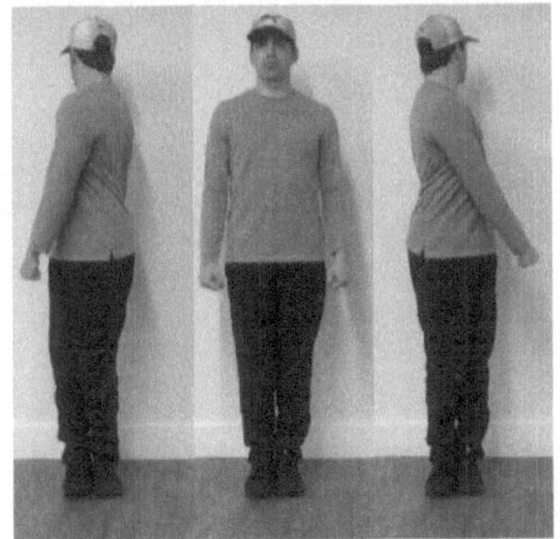

At the end of the book there will be a workout template with the 2- and 4-Day a week workout options.

As stated above in the warm-up section, it is encouraged to start from the phase 1 movements and then progress accordingly.

With the 12-Week Plan it is recommended to execute each phase for 4 weeks.

For example...

Week 1-4: Phase 1

Week 5-8: Phase 2

Week 9-12: Phase 3

There are also progressions (harder) and regressions (easier) for necessary exercises to help fit individual needs. If the individual cannot execute the progression with efficient form, then stick with the previous phase. It is important that we move efficiently, before progressing to the more advanced exercises.

*If there is any pain during exercises, refer out to a medical professional (Ex. Physical Therapist, Chiropractor, or potentially a trainer if the pain is being caused due to incorrect form). If the Bi-Lateral (both arms are being used at the same time) upper body exercises cause stress to the shoulders or neck try the single arm version, if that still bother's the shoulder, then reach out to a medical professional.

Upper Body

Movement - Vertical Push

Phase 1:

Quadruped Band Single Arm Eccentric Overhead Press

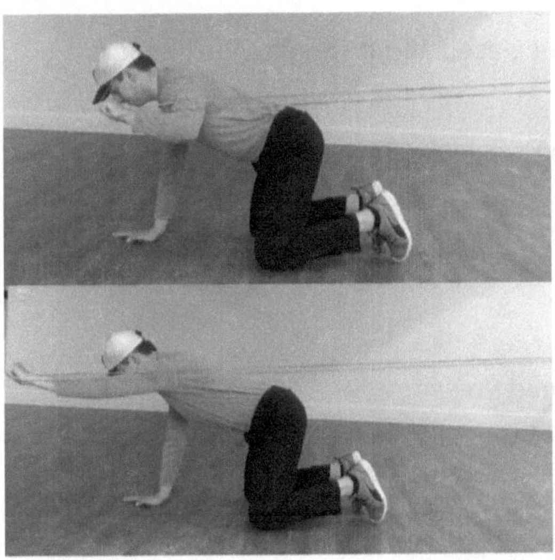

To Perform...

-In the quadruped position (Hands and Knees), place the knees directly below the hips and the hand on the ground directly below the shoulder

-The resistance band should be placed about shoulder height and attached to something sturdy

-Press the band overhead and take three seconds to bring it back to the beginning position

Phase 2:

Quadruped Single Arm Overhead Press

To Perform...

-In the quadruped position (Hands and Knees), place the knees directly below the hips and the hand on the ground directly below the shoulder

-The resistance band should be placed about shoulder height and attached to something sturdy

-Press the band overhead and then bring it back to the beginning position

Phase 3:

Push-Up Hold w/Band Overhead Press

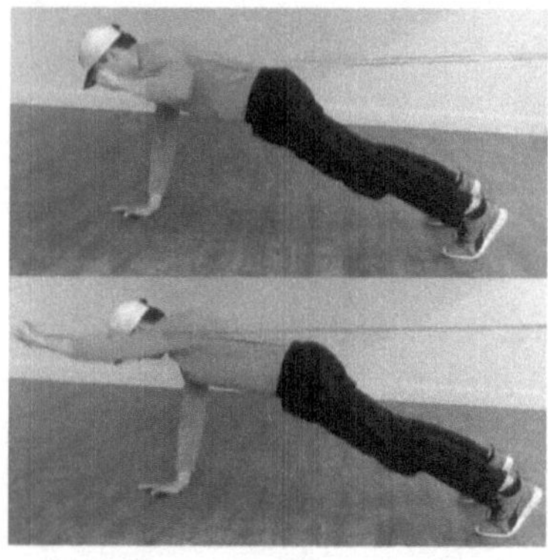

To Perform...

-In the push up position, dig the toes into the ground and place the hand on the ground directly below the shoulder

-The resistance band should be placed about shoulder height and attached to something sturdy

-Press the band overhead and bring it back to the beginning position

Movement - Horizontal Push

Phase 1:

Half-Kneeling Single Arm Band Press

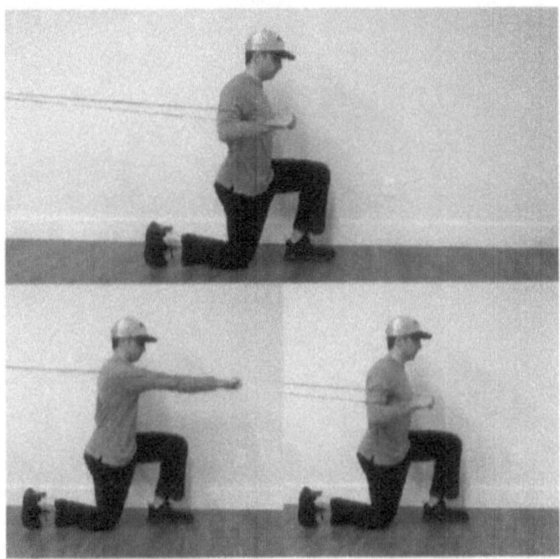

To Perform...

-Attach the band to something sturdy at about hip to shoulder height

-Grab the band with the hand that is opposite of the lead foot

-Grab the lead foot into the ground

-Press the band out and bring it back to the starting position from the half-kneeling position

Phase 2:

Standing Single Arm Press

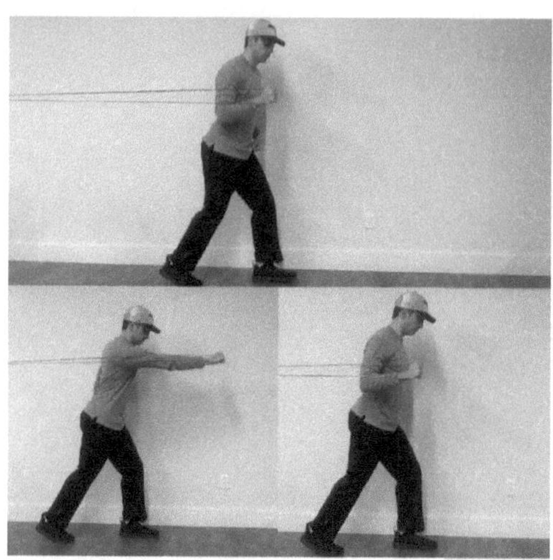

To Perform...

-Attach the band to something sturdy at about hip to shoulder height

-Grab the band with the hand that is opposite to the lead foot

-Starting from the split stance position proceed to grab the lead foot into the ground

-Then press the band out and bring it back to the starting position

*Most of the weight is on the lead foot

Phase 3:

Single Leg Single Arm Press

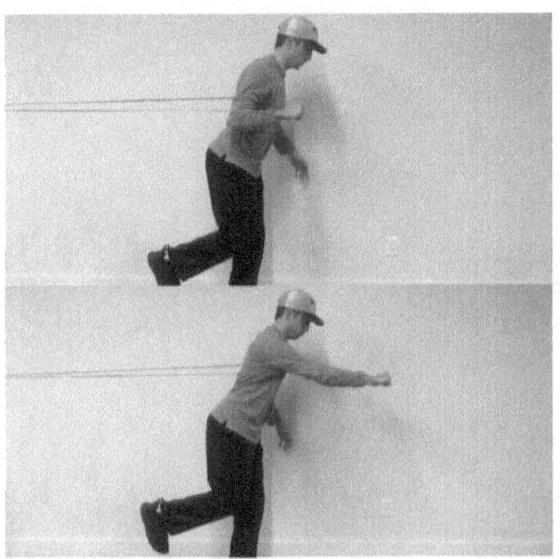

To Perform...

-Attach the band to something sturdy at about hip to shoulder height

-Grab the band with the hand of the foot that is on the ground

-Grab the foot into the ground

-Press the band out and bring it back to the starting position

Movement - Vertical Pull

Phase 1: Half-Kneeling Single Arm Vertical Pulldown

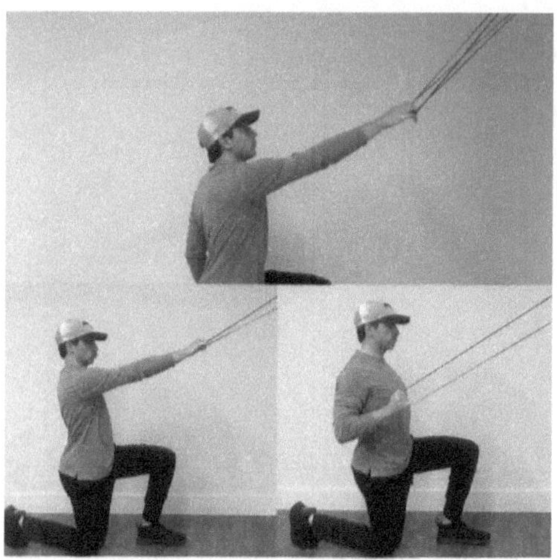

To Perform...

-Attach the band to something sturdy at a height well above the head

-From the half-kneeling position grip the band with the opposite hand of the lead foot

-Grab the lead foot into the ground

-Then proceed to pull the band in (Think: shoulder goes back with the elbow)

Phase 2: Half-Kneeling Vertical Pulldown

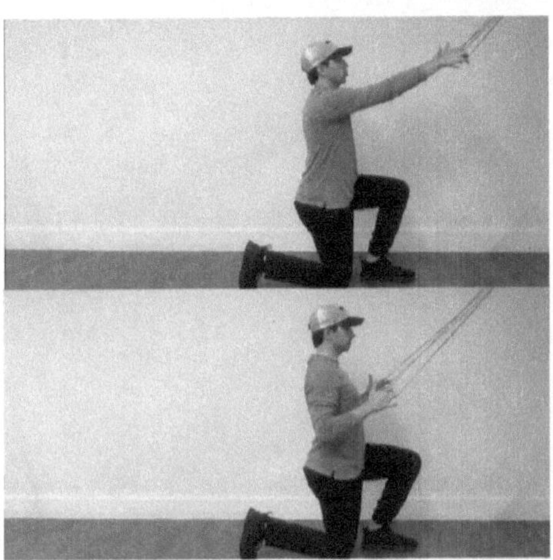

To Perform...

-Attach the band to something sturdy at a height well above the head (Use the strongest band possible, if the orange band is not enough resistance consider buying a stronger band or combining the orange and green band together for this exercise)

-From the half-kneeling position grab the band with the hands

-Grab the lead foot into the ground

-Then proceed to pull the band in (Think: shoulders go back with the elbows)

Phase 3: Half-Kneeling Speed Vertical Pulldown

To Perform...

-Repeat the steps from the Half-Kneeling Vertical Pulldown except pull the band in towards the chest as fast as possible (Slow on the way up)

Movement - Horizontal Pull

Phase 1:

Band Row w/Pause

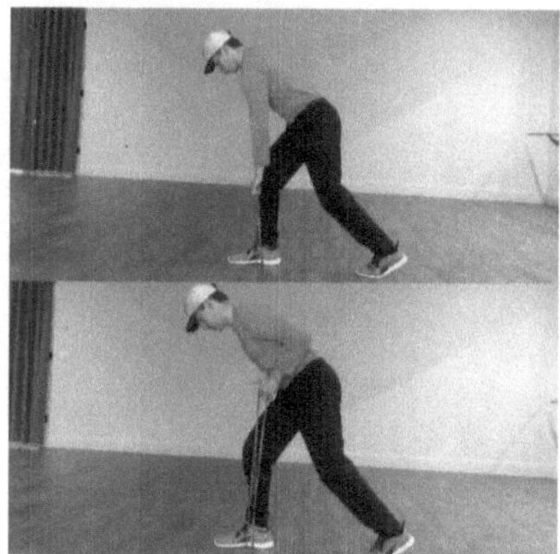

To Perform...

-Get into a split stance and place the band in the middle of the lead

foot

-Grab both sides of the resistance band with the hand opposite of

the lead foot

-Row towards the side of the chest and hold for 1-2 seconds

**Important to note, the shoulder that is pulling the band inward
should not tilt forward (Think: shoulder goes back with the elbow)

Phase 2:

Band Row

To Perform...

-Repeat steps from Phase 1 version listed above, except without a pause

**Important to note, the shoulder that is pulling the band inward
should not tilt forward (Think: shoulder goes back with the elbow)

Phase 3:

Band Row w/Speed

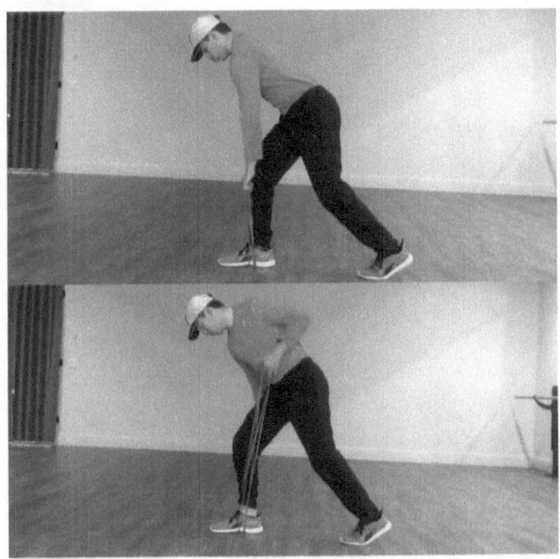

To Perform...

-Get into a split stance and place the band in the middle of the lead foot

-Grab both sides of the resistance band with the hand opposite of the lead foot

-Row towards the side of the chest at a fast rate and rotate the chest open to allow for increased speed

-Then proceed to slowly lower the band to the starting position

**Important to note, the shoulder that is pulling the band inward should not tilt forward (Think: shoulder goes back with the elbow)

**If the Standing Band Row is uncomfortable or painful, proceed to do this movement from the Half-Kneeling position as pictured below...

Phase 1: Half-Kneeling Band Row w/Pause

Phase 2: Half-Kneeling Band Row

Phase 3: Half-Kneeling Band Row w/Speed

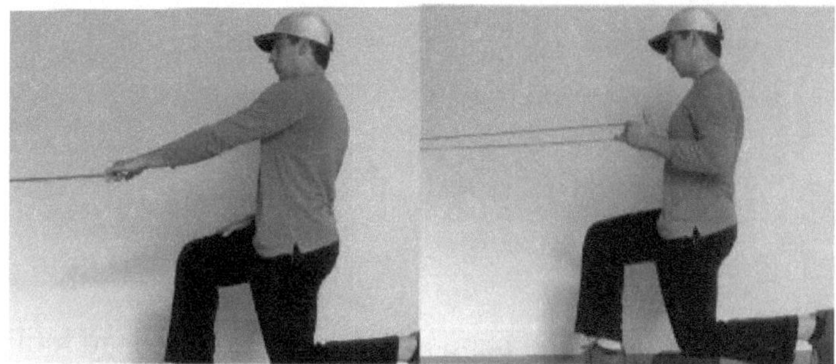

Lower Body

Movement - Single Leg Knee Dominant (Squat)

Phase 1:

Goblet Split Squat w/Band on Inside or w/Band on Outside of Knee

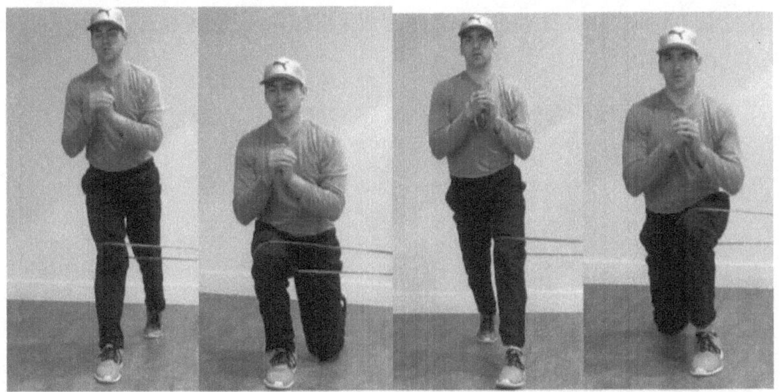

To perform...

-Place the resistance on something sturdy at the height of the knee

-Proceed to place the band around the inside or outside of the knee

-Make sure the back knee is directly below the hip and that the front knee is in between the lead heel and toe

-Grab the lead foot into the ground and push off through the lead leg to stand up

-Make sure most of the weight is distributed through the lead heel on the upward motion

How to choose which one....

*If the knee tends to bend inward when performing the split squat movement then put the band around the outside of the knee (left picture) to force the opposite muscles to activate

*If the knee tends to shift outward when performing the split squat movement then put the band around the inside of the knee (right picture) to force the opposite muscles to activate

Phase 2:

Pick One: Goblet Split Squat w/Band Pull, or Goblet Split Squat w/Band Pull to Chest

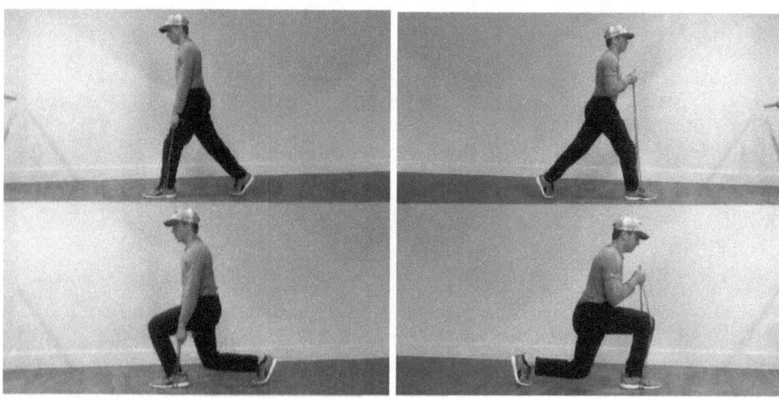

To Perform...

Goblet Split Squat w/Band Pull (Left)

-Place the resistance band under the middle of the lead foot

-Place each hand on the resistance band, one hand should be to the right of the lead leg and the other to the left of the lead leg

-From there grab the lead foot into the ground and push through the lead leg to stand up

-Make sure most of the weight is distributed through the lead heel on the upward motion

To Perform...

Goblet Split Squat w/Band Pull to Chest (Right)

-Place the resistance band under the middle of the lead foot

-Place each hand on the resistance band, one hand should be to the right of the lead leg and the other to the left of the lead leg

-Grip the band as if holding an ice cream cone and pull the band towards the center of the chest

-From there grab the lead foot into the ground and push through the lead leg to stand up

-Make sure most of the weight is distributed through the lead heel on the upward motion

Phase 3:

Rear Foot Elevated Split Squat w/Band (Optional)

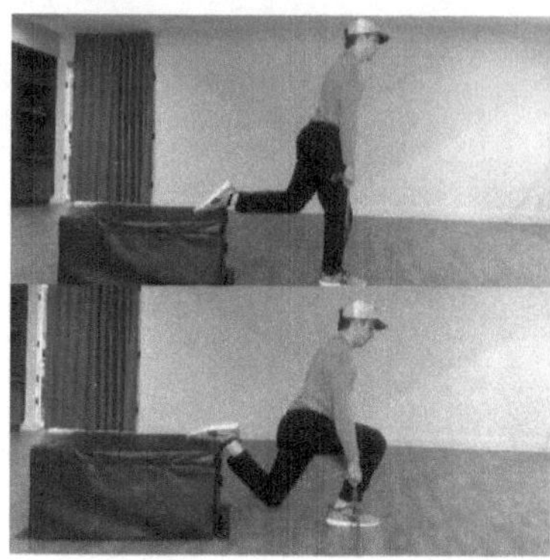

To Perform...

-Place the resistance band under the middle of the lead foot

-Place each hand on the resistance band, one hand should be to the right of the lead leg and the other to the left of the lead leg

-Then place the back foot on an elevated surface that is about knee height

-From there grab the lead foot into the ground and push through the lead leg to stand up

-Make sure most of the weight is distributed through the lead heel on the upward motion

Movement - Bilateral Knee Dominant (Squat)

Phase 1:

Goblet Squat w/Band Around Knees (BAK)

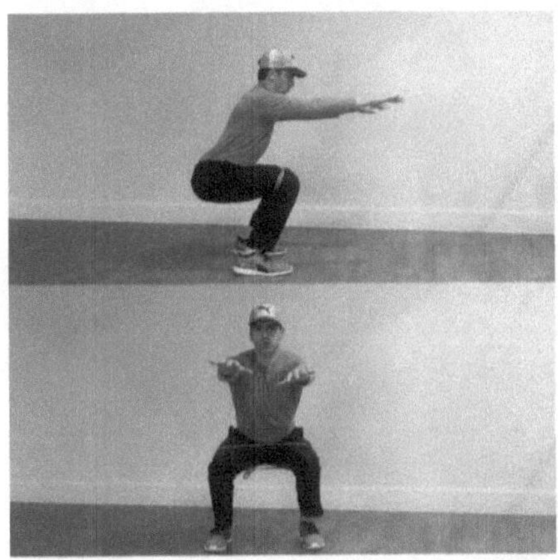

To Perform...

-Using a mini band or by tying the resistance band into a mini band, safely place the band around the knees

-Resist against the band so that the knees do not cave in

-Squat to parallel and stand back up

-It's important to note that placing the hands out in front, specifically on the downward motion will help for better balance

Phase 2:

Band Overhead Squat

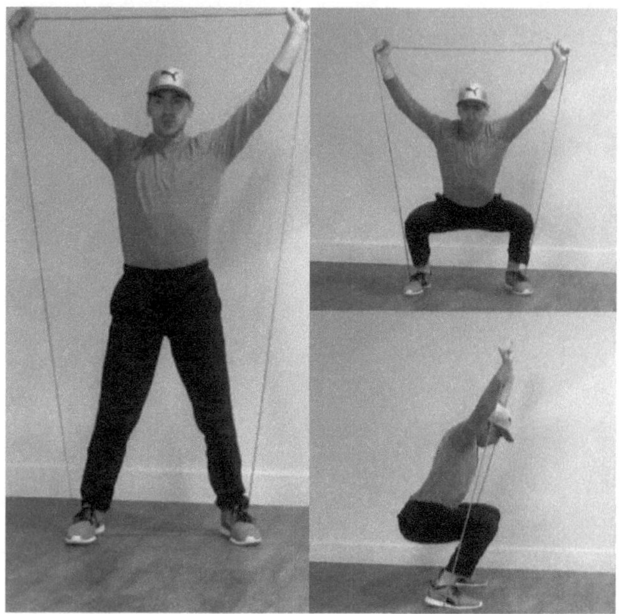

To Perform…

-Place the band under the feet and directly above the head.

-Grab the feet into the ground and squat down until the lower body (glute/hamstrings) is parallel with the floor.

-Then stand up. It's important to note that the hands stay up in the air the entire time.

Phase 3:

Band Overhead Squat w/Pause

To Perform...

-Repeat steps from Band Overhead Squat except pause for a second at the bottom

Movement - Single Leg Hip Dominant (Hip Hinge)

Phase 1:

Band Split Stance Single Leg RDL

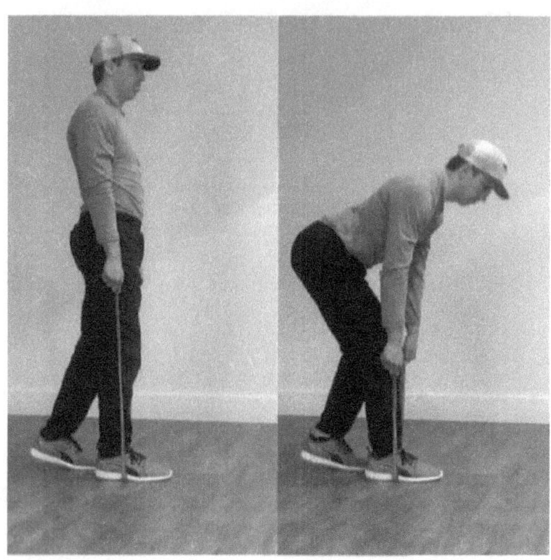

To Perform...

-Place the band under the middle of the lead foot

-Grab the band with necessary resistance (Grip lower on the band to make harder)

-Distribute most of the weight towards the heel of the lead foot and grab the lead foot into the ground

-Extend hip backwards, while maintaining a neutral spine

*Feel like the butt is going back-back-back-and then a little bit up at the end

Phase 2:

Band Split Stance w/3 Second Eccentric

To Perform...

-Repeat the same steps as the Band Split Stance Single Leg RDL except take three seconds on the downward hip hinge

Phase 3:

Band Split Stance w/Speed

To Perform...

-Repeat the same steps as the Band Split Stance Single Leg RDL except explode up, throughout the upward motion (Think: thrust the belt buckle forward)

Movement - Bilateral Hip Dominant (Hip Hinge)

Phase 1:

Band RDL

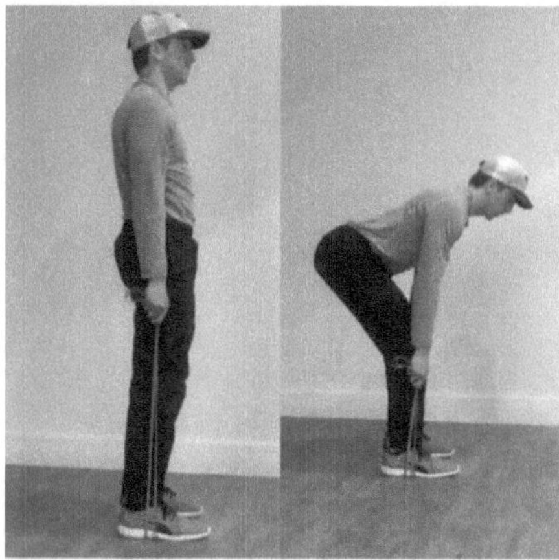

To Perform...

-Place the resistance band under the middle of the feet

-Place each hand on the resistance band, one hand should be to the right of the legs and the other hand to the left of the legs

-From there, grab the feet into the ground and push through the floor with most of the weight towards the heels and stand up tall

Phase 2:

Band RDL w/3 Second Eccentric

To Perform...

-Repeat the same steps as the Band RDL but take 3 seconds on the downward motion.

Phase 3:

Band RDL w/Speed

-Repeat the same steps as the Band RDL but explode up, throughout the upward motion. (Think: thrust the belt buckle forward)

Core

Movement - Anti-Lateral Flexion

Phase 1:

Half-Kneeling Anti-Lateral Flexion

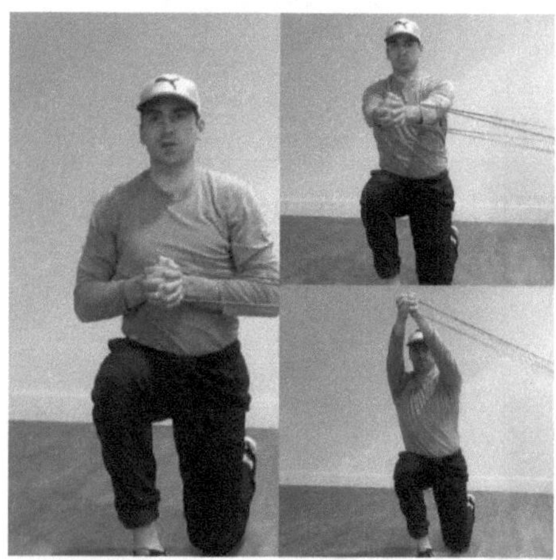

To Perform…

-Place the band against something sturdy at chest height

-Place the inside hand around the band and then overlap or interlock the opposing hand

-From the half-kneeling position, proceed to tighten the stomach (as if taking a punch), grab the lead foot into the ground, and press the band forward by straightening the arms

-Proceed to raise the arms up as high as possible, while keeping the arms straight

-Then lower down and bring the band back towards the chest

Phase 2:

Isometric Anti-Lateral Flexion

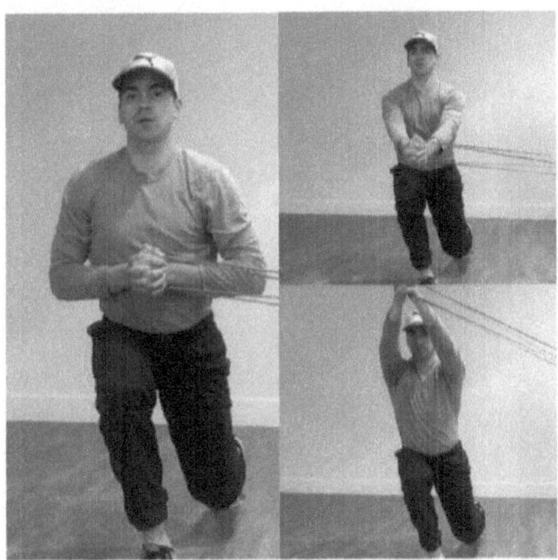

To Perform...

-Place the band against something sturdy at chest height

-Place the inside hand around the band and then overlap or interlock the opposing hand

-From the half-kneeling position, ensure that the back toes are firm into the ground and lift the back knee 1-3 inches off the ground

-Proceed to tighten the stomach (as if taking a punch), grab the lead foot into the ground, and press the band forward by straightening the arms

-Proceed to raise the arms up as high as possible, while keeping the arms straight

-Then lower down and bring the band back towards the chest

Phase 3:

Standing Anti-Lateral Flexion

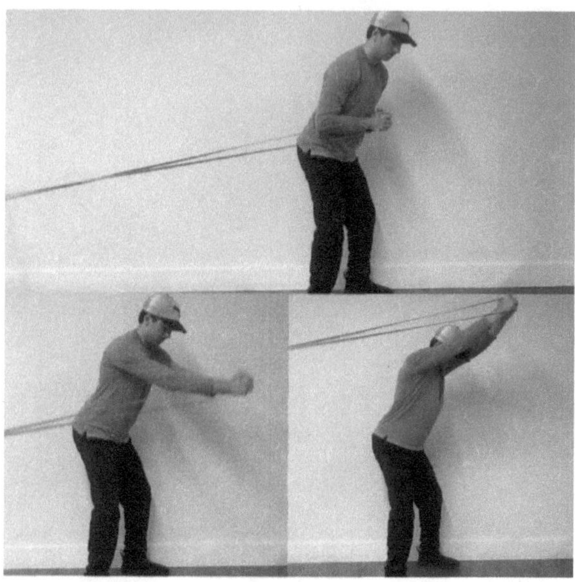

To Perform...

-Place the band against something sturdy at waist-chest height

-Place the inside hand around the band and then overlap or interlock the opposing hand

-From the standing position, proceed to tighten the stomach (as if taking a punch), grab the feet into the ground, and press the band forward by straightening the arms

-Proceed to raise the arms up as high as possible, while keeping the arms straight

-Then lower the arms down and bring the band back towards the chest

Movement - Anti-Rotation

Phase 1:

Half-Kneeling Anti-Rotation Press

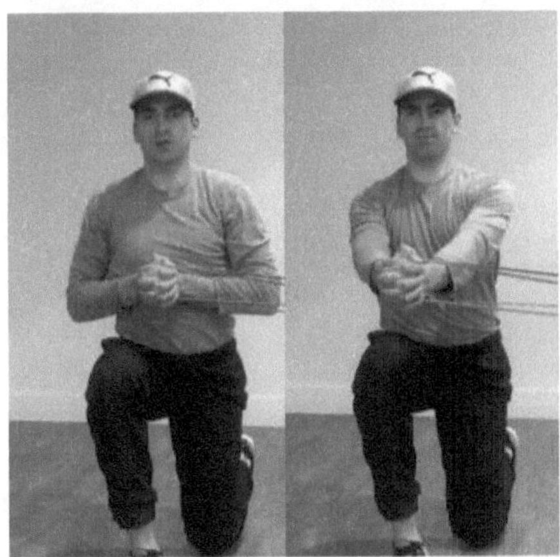

To Perform...

-Place the band against something sturdy at chest height

-Place the inside hand around the band and then overlap or interlock the opposing hand

-From the half-kneeling position, proceed to tighten the stomach (as if taking a punch), grab the lead foot into the ground, and press the band forward by straightening the arms

Phase 2:

Standing Anti-Rotation Press w/Hold

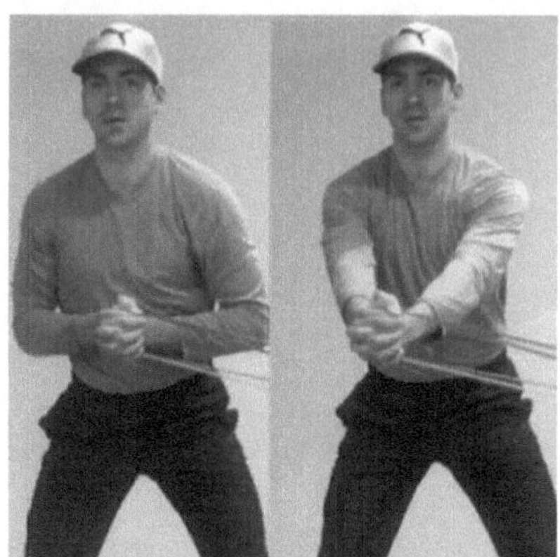

To Perform...

-Place the band against something sturdy at waist to chest height

-Place the inside hand around the band and then overlap or interlock the opposing hand

-From the standing position, proceed to tighten the stomach (as if taking a punch), grab the feet into the ground, and press the band forward by straightening the arms

-Hold for prescribed amount of time

Phase 3:

Standing Anti-Rotation Press

To Perform...

-Repeat steps from the standing anti-rotation press w/hold, except without the hold

Movement - Chop/Lift

Phase 1:

Half-Kneeling Lift w/Band

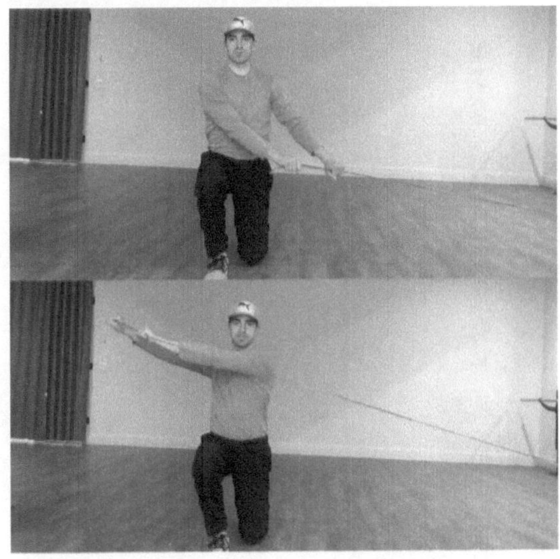

To Perform...

-Get into the half-kneeling position

-Attach the band to something sturdy and as close to the ground as possible

-Grip the band as if riding a motorcycle (shoulder width and palms toward the ground)

-Keeping the arms straight and lower body stable, grab the lead foot into the ground, and lift the band upward and across the body

**Important to note, rotation will happen with the upper body but should be limited

Phase 2:

Standing Lift w/Band

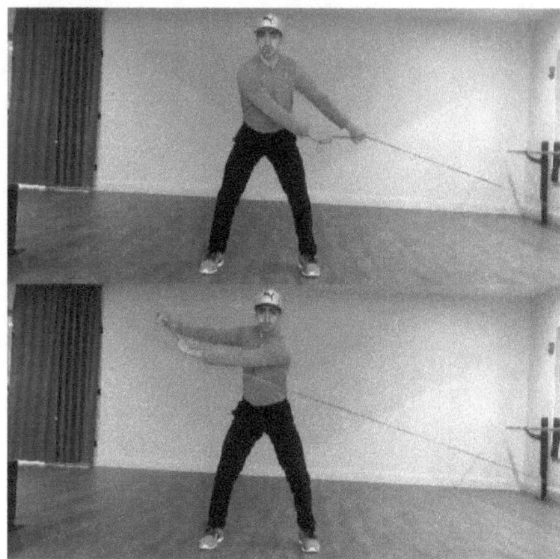

To Perform…

-Get into an athletic stance

-Attach the band to something sturdy and as close to the ground as possible

-Grip the band as if riding a motorcycle (shoulder width and palms toward the ground)

-Keeping the arms straight and lower body stable, grab the feet into the ground, and lift the band upward and across the body

**Important to note, rotation will happen with the upper body but should be limited

Phase 3:

Speed Lift w/Band

To Perform…

-Repeat steps from the standing lift except add as much speed as possible on the upward motion

Phase 1:

Half-Kneeling Chop w/Band

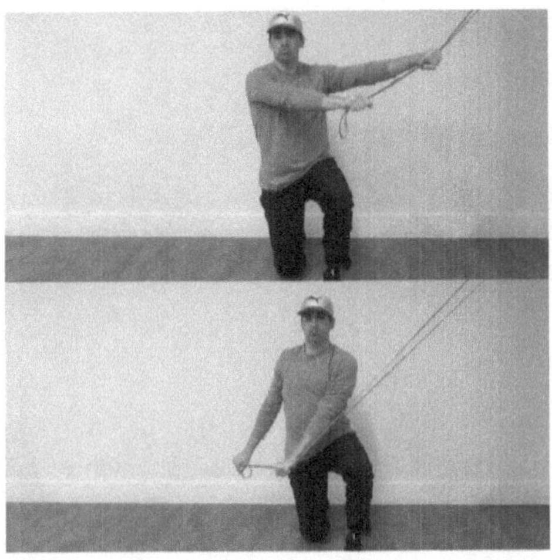

To Perform...

-Get into the half-kneeling position

-Attach the band to something sturdy and well above the height of the head

-Grip the band as if riding a motorcycle (shoulder width and palms toward the ground)

-Keeping the arms straight and lower body stable, grab the lead foot into the ground, and pull the band downward and across the body

**Important to note, rotation will happen with the upper body but should be limited

Phase 2:

Standing Chop w/Band

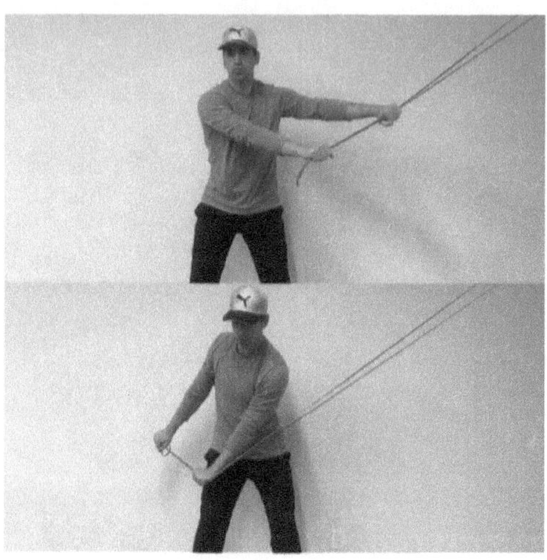

To Perform...

-Attach the band to something sturdy and well above the height of the head

-From the standing position grip the band as if riding a motorcycle (shoulder width and palms toward the ground)

-Keeping the arms straight and lower body stable, grip the feet into the ground, and pull the band downward and across the body

**Important to note, rotation will happen with the upper body but should be limited

Phase 3:

Speed Chop w/Band

To Perform...

-Repeat the steps for the standing chop except add some speed on the downward motion

Accessory

Calves/Tib Anterior

Phase 1:

Seated Tib Anterior

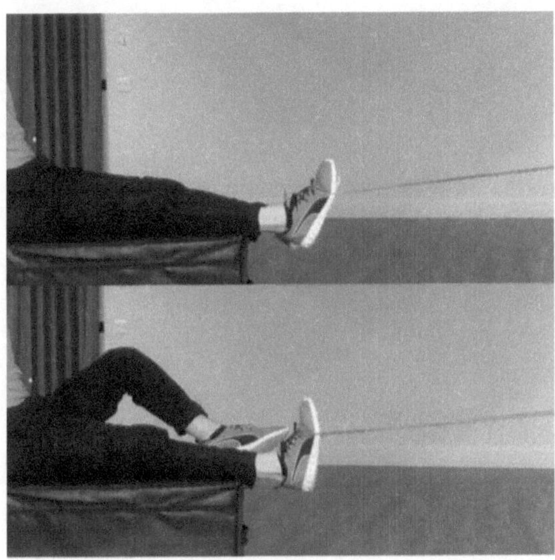

To Perform…

-From the seated position, place the foot just off the bench, box, bed, or anything that is sturdy and will allow the leg to stay straight

-Place the band about 2/3's of the way up the foot, with the band being on the shoelace side and attached to something sturdy

-Flex the toes towards the chest and then extend away

Phase 2:

Calf Raise w/3 Second Eccentric

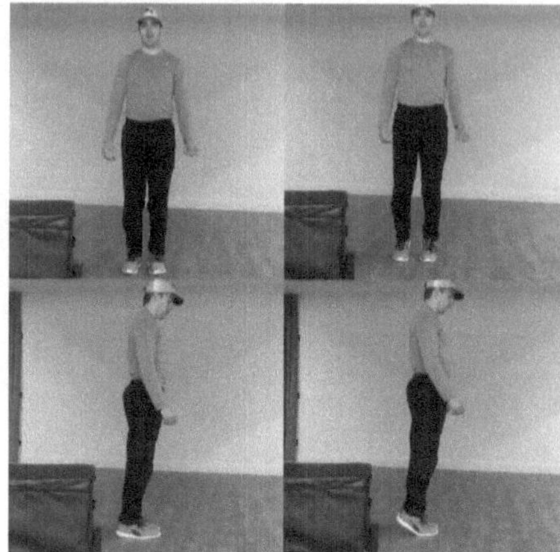

To Perform...

-Maintain an upright position with the body

-If necessary, place hand(s) on a wall to help maintain balance

-Raise the heels up as high as possible while maintaining balance

-Take three seconds to lower the heels back to the ground

Phase 3:

Single Leg Calf Raise w/Single Leg Eccentric

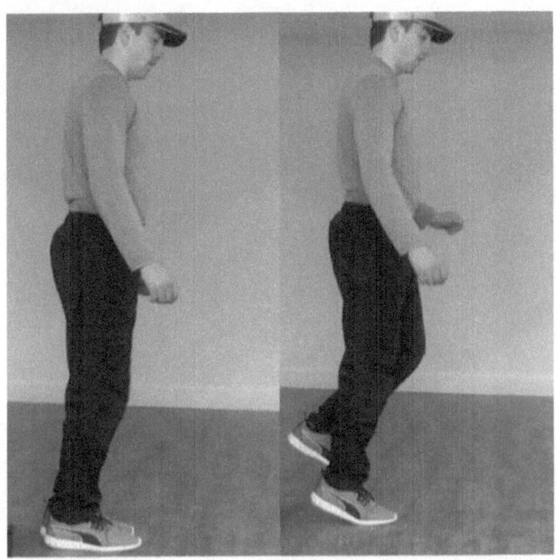

To Perform...

-Repeat steps from standing calf raise except on one leg

-If necessary, place hand(s) on a wall to help maintain balance

-Take three seconds to lower the heels back to the ground

Phase 1:

Seated Calf Raise w/Band

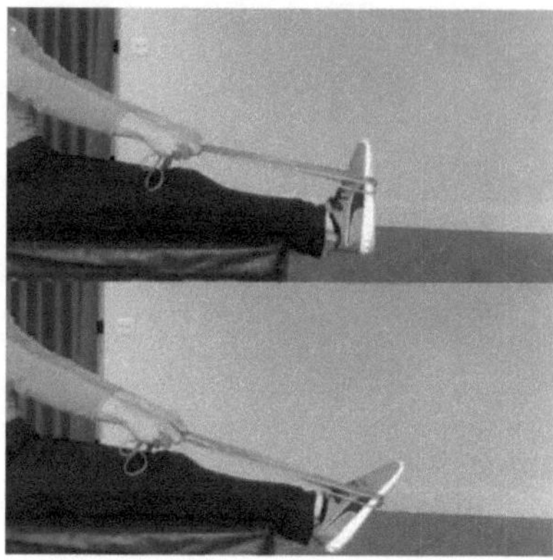

To Perform…

-From the seated position, place the foot just off the bench, box, bed, or anything else that is sturdy and will allow the leg to stay straight

-Place the band about 2/3's of the way up the foot

-Pull the band towards the chest

-Proceed to flex the toes up toward the body and then extend away

Phase 2:

Standing Calf Raise

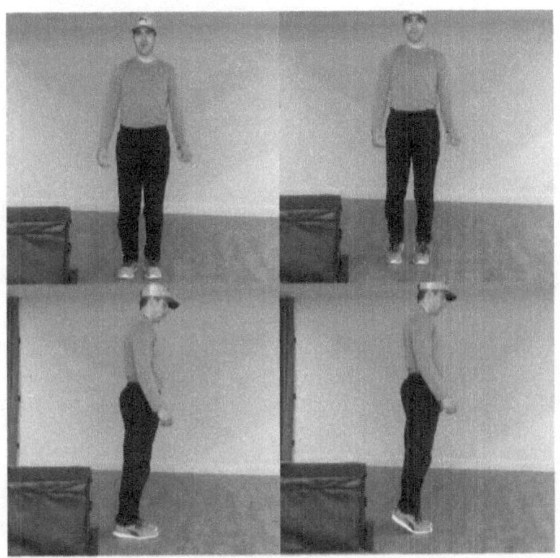

To Perform...

-Maintain an upright position with the body

-Raise the heels up as high as possible while maintaining balance

Phase 3:

Single Leg Standing Calf Raise

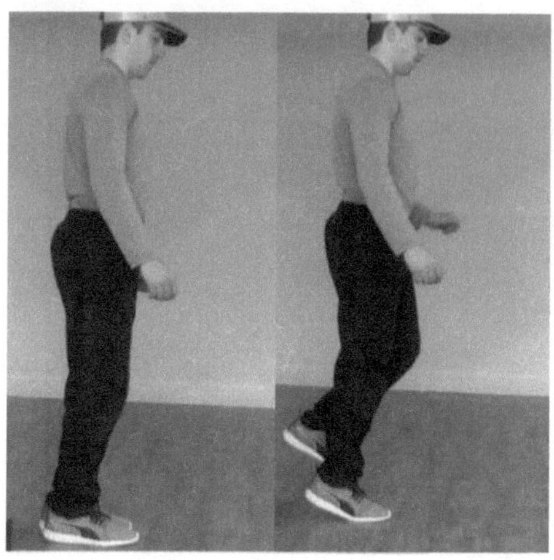

To Perform...

-Repeat steps from standing calf raise except on one leg

-If necessary, place hand on a wall to help maintain balance

Rotator Cuff

Phase 1:

Band No Money's

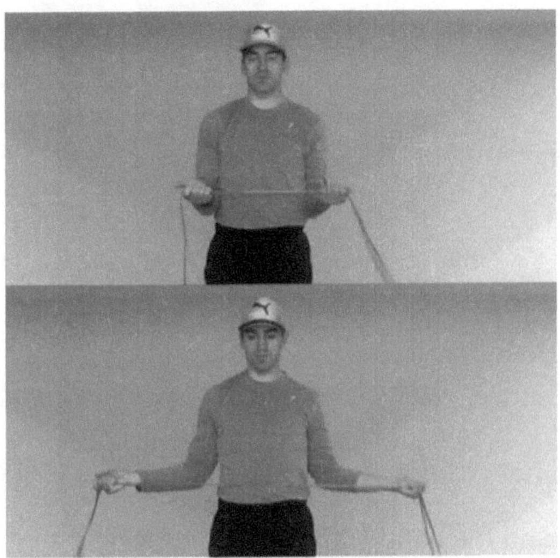

To Perform...

-Ensure the shoulders are not tilting forward

-Grip the feet into the ground and the band at a width that is comfortable to the right resistance for the individual

-Keep the elbows close to the side of the body and pull the hands back as far as possible

-Keep elbows and wrist at the same level the entire time

Phase 2:

Band Pullaparts

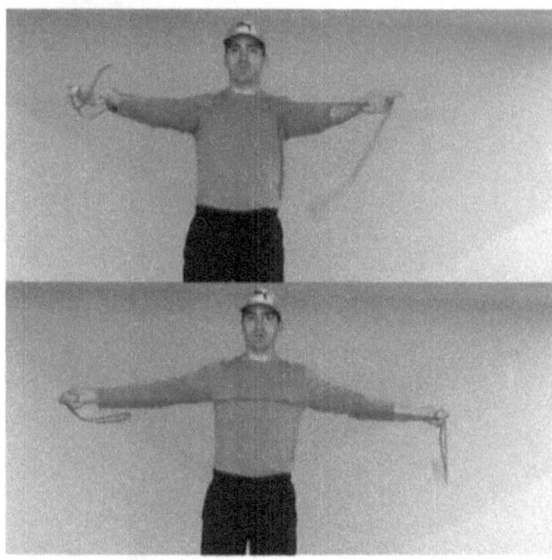

To Perform…

-Ensure that the shoulders are not tilting forward

-Grip the feet into the ground and the band with the palms facing the sky

-Adjust the hands appropriate to the necessary resistance

-Keep the arms straight and pull the band backwards

Phase 3:

Band Pullaparts + Band No Money's

To Perform…

-Proceed to execute the band pullaparts for the prescribed amount of reps and then perform the band no money's next

Phase 1:

Single Arm Band No Money's

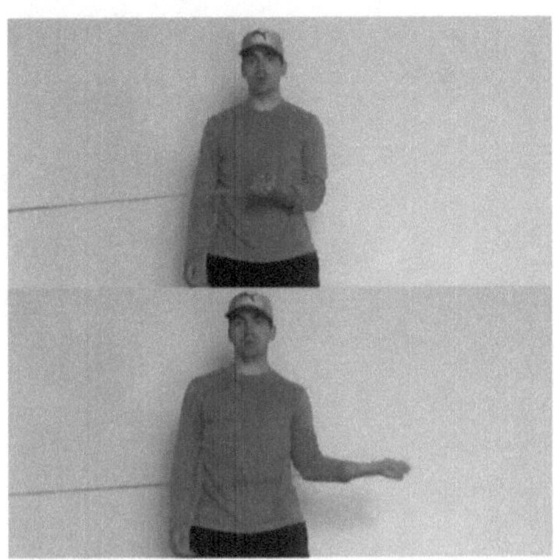

To Perform...

-Place the palm to the sky and grab the feet into the ground

-Keeping the elbow fairly close to the side of the abdomen for the moving arm

-Rotate the arm and band away from the body

Phase 2:

Single Arm Band Pullaparts

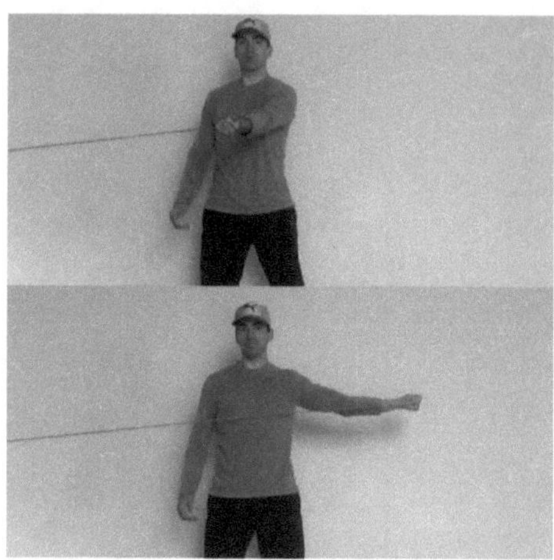

To Perform...

-Place the palm up to the sky and grab the feet into the ground

-Keep the arm gripping the band fairly straight

-Pull the band away from the body

-Feel like the shoulder is doing most of the work

Phase 3:

Single Arm Band Pullaparts + Single Arm Band No Money's

To Perform...

-Proceed to execute the single arm band pullaparts for the prescribed amount of reps and then perform the single arm band no money's next

Chapter 6: Conditioning

The main goal behind conditioning with golfers is to be able to play the last hole with as much energy as the first hole, along with the rest of the holes in between. During a round of golf there are many challenges that affect golfer's stamina levels. These challenges include:

- Repetitively swinging a golf club
- Maintaining posture throughout the swing
- Walking up and down hills
- Maintaining energy levels

Conditioning will help target improvements in all four of these areas...

Below is a list of various ways to add conditioning into the workouts. Considering everyone is different, choose the one that works best for the individual and their specific goals.

- For someone looking to improve swing speed, the **Super Speed swing protocol** will most likely be the best fit.
- For someone with knees that have had some wear and tear and has access to a bike (either stationary or moving), the **biking protocol** will most likely be the best fit.
- For someone who wants to improve endurance throughout the round, the walking or running protocol will most likely be the best fit.
- For someone who has limited space and equipment the **skiers protocol** will most likely be a great fit.

Lower Body - Conditioning

Option 1 – Bikes

Phase 1:

30 Seconds Medium-Fast/30 Seconds Slow

Phase 2:

15 Seconds Fast/30 Seconds Slow

Phase 3:

10 Seconds Fast/20 Seconds Slow

Option 2 – Running/Walking (Use a treadmill or anywhere you can run/walk)

Phase 1:

30 Seconds Slow or Off (if running)/30 Seconds Medium/Fast (Suggested Incline of 10%)

Phase 2:

15 Seconds Fast/30 Seconds Slow or Off (if running) (Suggested Incline of 10%)

Phase 3:

10 Seconds Fast/20 Seconds Slow or Off (if running) (Recommended Incline of 10%)

Upper Body - Conditioning

Option 1 - Super Speed Training

Phase 1 – Level 1 Protocol

Phase 2 – Level 1 Protocol for the first 2 weeks & Level 2 Protocol for the last 2 weeks

Phase 3 – Level 2 Protocol

This is the exact protocol, from SuperSpeed Golf. For more on how to keep progressing with the SuperSpeed sticks after the 12-Week Program, please visit their website at...

https://superspeedgolf.com/

Upper Body - Conditioning

Option 1 - Super Speed Training

Level 1 - Protocol

| LEVEL 1 | | | |
POSITION	LIGHT	MEDIUM	HEAVY
1 Normal	3 Each Side	3 Each Side	3 Each Side
2 Step-Change	3 Each Side	3 Each Side	3 Each Side
3 Normal	3 Dominant		

Level 2 – Protocol

| LEVEL 2 | | | |
POSITION	LIGHT	MEDIUM	HEAVY
1 Normal	3 Each Side	3 Each Side	3 Each Side
2 Kneeling	3 Each Side	3 Each Side	3 Each Side
3 Step-Change	3 Each Side	3 Each Side	3 Each Side
4 Normal	3 Dominant		

Option 2 - Skiers w/Superflex

Phase 1:

30 Seconds fast to medium/30 Seconds Rest

Phase 2:

15 Seconds fast/30 Seconds Rest

Phase 3:

10 Seconds fast/20 Seconds Rest

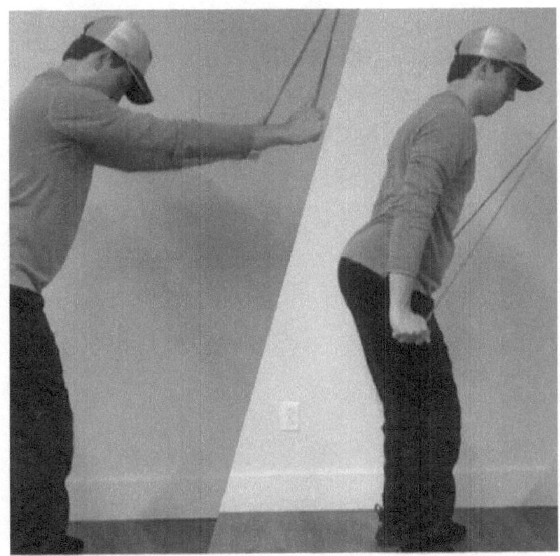

To Perform...

-Pull the band downward towards the side pockets

-Perform as fast as possible on the downward motion

Chapter 7: The Team Approach

It's important to note that the purpose of "The Ultimate In-Home Golf Fitness Program" is to improve distance, durability, and flexibility to give golfers an increased potential to play more efficiently and effectively. However, there are many other components in golf that need to be touched on when trying to lower scores consistently. With the correct team, every area towards improvement can be addressed and worked on. Building an effective team will give golfers the best chance to succeed at all levels.

In 2016, I heard from one of Justin Rose's coaches that there were around 13-14 members on his team. Most golfers do not need that many people on their team. But, to simplify the team approach I've broken it down into 4 categories.

Which include the....

- Swing Coach
- Fitness Professional
- Medical Professional
- Mental Coach

Swing Coach:

They are in charge of the golf swing technique, course management, and have many other duties that involve lowering the players scores.

The most important credential when looking for a swing coach would be, "can they get the golfer to hit the ball where they want to". If not, then they better have a plan in place to allow that to happen.

A swing coach should be able to help the golfer...

1.) Hit the ball far enough to play the course effectively
2.) Control the direction of the shot
3.) Help the golfer make solid contact

With consistent contact, control, and distance golfers are most likely going to improve their game. Keep it simple and find a coach who can help! When looking for a swing coach, typically look for a **PGA Teaching Professional, PGA Professional** who teaches **over 15 lessons a week**, or a **Teaching Professional** who **teaches** for a **living**.

Fitness Professional:

The fitness professional is in charge of keeping the golfer strong, moving well, and developing an injury prevention strategy. Nutrition can also be outsourced but the fitness professional should be able to provide some guidance on this topic as well.

When looking for a fitness professional it is important to find someone who has a **structured evaluation**. Typically, I recommend people find a professional who is Functional Movement Screen (FMS) certified. This screen helps fitness professionals **design a plan** structured around what the individual can or cannot do.

There are also many great training certifications to look for in fitness professionals such as the Certified Strength and Conditioning Specialist (CSCS), Titleist Performance Institute Level 2 or 3 Certified tracks, and Certified Functional Strength Coach Level 2 Certified (CFSC-2).

When looking for nutrition coaching the main certification to look for is Precision Nutrition Level 1 or 2 (PN-1, PN-2). Precision Nutrition has a simple and effective system to help live an improved quality of life through improving different nutritional habits over time.

However, **it is important** to find someone with **experience** and a **plan to help you reach your specific goals**.

Medical Professional:

The medical professional is in charge of soft tissue work, any source of pain or injury, and may also work with the fitness professional on an injury prevention plan.

When looking for a medical professional, it is typically better **to look and listen for referrals first**. The main credential to look for is the **Selective Functional Movement Assessment (SFMA)**. This is a system that allows the medical professional to get to the bottom of what the issue is.

Medical professional may also refer out to trusted Orthopedic Doctors, Physicians, and Registered Dietitians depending on what the issue is.

Mental Coach:

The mental coach is in charge of getting the golfers **mind right** and helping them **reach their true potential**. The mental coach can work with the player individually or with both players and coaches.

Chapter 8: Getting Started

The purpose of this book is to present a progressive fitness program that can be done with minimal equipment, in a short period of time, and give golfers the potential to play longer and score lower.

Overall, we were able to simplify the golf swing and relate it into fitness terminology, design a basic program (Foam Roll, Joint-By-Joint Warm-Up, Strength, and Conditioning), and explain the importance of the team approach.

Details included everything from priming mobility, to gaining the proper stability in the joints to achieve and maintain a healthy golf swing over time, and also a plan showing golfer's how to build a foundation of strength to give them the potential to achieve improved results.

Always feel free to contact me or your local TPI Certified Golf, Medical, or Fitness Professional for further advice and understanding as well.

Below are links to all the **equipment** you will need for the program……

    1.) Super Speed Golf Sticks –
        https://superspeedgolf.com/

        Discount Code – bggandf

    2.) Perform Better 18" Foam Roller –
        https://www.performbetter.com/

    3.) The Home Golf Fitness Kit: SuperFlex Resistance Bands, Handles, and Clips –
        https://www.superflexfitness.com/
        Click – Packages
        Scroll Down – Home Golf Fitness Package

        Discount Code: Golf Kit

<u>Order of the Workouts</u>

1.) **Foam Roll: *Optional* 5-10 minutes**
    -Roll for necessary amount.
2.) **Joint-By-Joint Warm-Up: 5-10 minutes**
    -Perform one round for each exercise listed before proceeding to the warm-up circuit.
3.) **Movement Warm-Up (Warm-Up Circuit): 10 minutes**
    -Perform one round, then repeat for a total of two rounds before proceeding to strength training.
4.) **Strength Training: 15-20 minutes**
    -Perform exercises in the order listed for the necessary amount of rounds. The two day program has two different circuits separated by the bold lines. While the four day program has one circuit.
5.) **Conditioning: 5-10 minutes**
    -Perform at the end for the prescribed amount. Once this is finished the workout is complete.

<u>The 12-Week Program Spreadsheets</u>

Below is a list of spreadsheets for "The Ultimate In-Home Golf Fitness Program". It is recommended to have this nearby for a more efficient and time productive workout. When finished, mark off the day that was completed.

To help clear up any confusion with the wording on the spreadsheets here are some abbreviations and explanations to potential questions.

HK – Half Kneeling

Quad – Quadruped Position (On hands and knees)

Supine – Laying on the Back

Reps – Amount of Repetitions to perform

Ea. – Reps Each Side

SL – Single Leg

SA – Single Arm

SLDL – Single Leg Deadlift

RDL – Romanian Deadlift

OH – Overhead

The Bold Lines – Represent a circuit, therefore all exercises should be performed in order. Once completed move on to the next section.

3x8 – Means 3 Sets and 8 Repetitions for each of those set

Rep Stack – If there is one exercise followed by a stack of reps

Ex.) 8

8

8

Then that would mean 3 Sets of 8 Repetitions as well.

Name:

12 Week Progressive Golf Performance Program

Two Day - Phase 1

Goals:

1.) Build A Foundation of Strength

Foam Roll:

Foam Roll / Mobility	Reps
Ankle: Supine Ankle Flexion & Extension + Supine Ankle Windshield Wipers	1x8 Ea.
Knee: Supine Knee Flexion/Extension	5 Sec. Holds (x2 Ea. Side)
Hip Extension/Flexion: Alt. Leg Lowers	1x8 Ea.
Hip Internal/External: Supine Hip Circles or Passive Straight Leg Twist	1x5 Ea.
Lower Back: Supine Pelvic Tilts	1x8 Ea.
T-Spine: Supine Arm Bar (Progression: Add a Kettlebell or Dumbbell)	1x8 Ea.
Scapula: Supine Floor Slides + Supine Arm Reaches	1x6 Ea.
Shoulder: *Targeted Above in a Two-in-One Exercises - Supine Arm Bar w/Internal and External Rotation (Progression: Add a Kettlebell or Dumbbell)	
Wrist/Elbow: Supine Wrist Press Ups + Ulnar and Radial Wrist Flexion + Supine Wrist Flexion and Extension	1x6 Ea.
Neck: Supine Neck Flexion & Extension + Supine Neck Side to Side Rotations	1x3 Ea.

Day 1 - Warm-Up Circuit:	Week 1	Reps	Week 2	Reps	Week 3	Reps	Week 4	Reps
Jump Squats		2x8		2x8		2x8		2x8
Push-Up Hold		2x8 Br.		2x8 Br.		2x8 Br.		2x8 Br.
SL Cook Hip Lift		2x8 Ea.		2x8 Ea.		2x8 Ea.		2x8 Ea.
Bird Dogs		2x6 Ea.		2x6 Ea.		2x6 Ea.		2x6 Ea.

Day 1 - Lower Body Workout	Week 1	Reps	Week 2	Reps	Week 3	Reps	Week 4	Reps
Goblet Squat w/BAK		8		8		8		8
		8		8		8		8
		8		8		8		8
Quadruped w/Band Eccentric OH Press		8 Ea.		8 Ea.		8 Ea.		8 Ea.
		8 Ea.		8 Ea.		8 Ea.		8 Ea.
		8 Ea.		8 Ea.		8 Ea.		8 Ea.
HK Chop or Lift w/Band (Pick One)		3x8 Ea.		3x8 Ea.		3x8 Ea.		3x8 Ea.
HK SA Band Vertical Pulldown		8 Ea.		8 Ea.		8 Ea.		8 Ea.
		8 Ea.		8 Ea.		8 Ea.		8 Ea.
		8 Ea.		8 Ea.		8 Ea.		8 Ea.
Band Split Stance SL RDL		8 Ea.		8 Ea.		8 Ea.		8 Ea.
		8 Ea.		8 Ea.		8 Ea.		8 Ea.
		8 Ea.		8 Ea.		8 Ea.		8 Ea.
Seated Tib Anterior		3x8 Ea.		3x8 Ea.		3x8 Ea.		3x8 Ea.

Day 1 - Conditioning: Bikes, Running, or Walking - 30 Seconds Medium-Fast/30 Seconds Rest or Slow [Week - 1 (x6), 2 (x6), 3 (x8), 4 (x8)]

Day 2 - Warm-Up Circuit:	Week 1	Reps	Week 2	Reps	Week 3	Reps	Week 4	Reps
Half-Kneeling Rotational Throw w/Band		2x6 Ea.		2x6 Ea.		2x6 Ea.		2x6 Ea.
Side Plank from Knees		2x8 Ea.		2x8 Ea.		2x8 Ea.		2x8 Ea.
Assisted Lateral Lunge w/Band		2x6 Ea.		2x6 Ea.		2x6 Ea.		2x6 Ea.
Single Leg Balance		2x15 Sec. Ea.		2x15 Sec. Ea.		2x15 Sec. Ea.		2x15 Sec. Ea.

Day 2 - Upper Body Workout	Week 1	Reps	Week 2	Reps	Week 3	Reps	Week 4	Reps
Band RDL		10		10		10		10
		10		10		10		10
		10		10		10		10
Band Row w/Pause		8 Ea.		8 Ea.		8 Ea.		8 Ea.
		8 Ea.		8 Ea.		8 Ea.		8 Ea.
		8 Ea.		8 Ea.		8 Ea.		8 Ea.
Band No Money's (Optional: Single Arm)		3x10 Ea.		3x10 Ea.		3x10 Ea.		3x10 Ea.
HK SA Press		8 Ea.		8 Ea.		8 Ea.		8 Ea.
		8 Ea.		8 Ea.		8 Ea.		8 Ea.
		8 Ea.		8 Ea.		8 Ea.		8 Ea.
Goblet Split Squat w/Band on Inside or Outside of Knee		8 Ea.		8 Ea.		8 Ea.		8 Ea.
		8 Ea.		8 Ea.		8 Ea.		8 Ea.
		8 Ea.		8 Ea.		8 Ea.		8 Ea.
Seated Calf Raise w/Band		3x8 Ea.		3x8 Ea.		3x8 Ea.		3x8 Ea.

Day 2 - Conditioning: Super Speed Sticks (Phase 1- See Conditioning Section in Book for Details)

Name:

12 Week Progressive Golf Performance Program

Two Day - Phase 2

Goals:

1.) Build A Foundation of Strength

Foam Roll:

Day 1	Reps		Day 2	Reps
Ankle: HK Ankle Dorso-Flexion + HK Side to Side Ankle Dorso-Flexion	1x8 Ea.		Hip Flexion/Extension: Quadruped Hip Extension	1x8 Ea.
Knee: Quadruped Single Leg Extension	1x8 Ea.		Hip Internal/External: Quadruped Hip Circles	1x5 Ea.
			Lower Back: Cat & Camels	1x8 Ea.
			T-Spine: Quadruped T-Spine Ext. Rotation (Progression: HK T-Spine Rotations)	1x8 Ea.
			Scapula: Half-Kneeling Single Arm Reach + Half-Kneeling Elevation and Depression	1x6 Ea.
			Shoulder: Half-Kneeling Arm Circle (Both forward and backward)	1x3 Ea.
			Wrist/Elbow: Quadruped Wrist Mobs (Flexion & Extension)	1x6 Ea.
			Neck: Quadruped Side to Side w/Chin to Sternum or Tall-Kneeling Side to Side Twist w/Chin to Sternum	1x3 Ea.

Day 1 - Warm-Up Circuit

	Week 1	Reps	Week 2	Reps	Week 3	Reps	Week 4	Reps
Single Leg Jump Squat w/Bilateral Landing		2x4 Ea.		2x4 Ea.		2x4 Ea.		2x4 Ea.
Plank		2x8 Br.		2x8 Br.		2x8 Br.		2x8 Br.
SL Cook Hip Lift w/Hold (10 Sec.)		2x3 Ea.		2x3 Ea.		2x3 Ea.		2x3 Ea.
Bird Dogs Holds (5 Sec. Ea.)		2x3 Ea.		2x3 Ea.		2x3 Ea.		2x3 Ea.

Day 2 - Warm-Up Circuit

	Week 1	Reps	Week 2	Reps	Week 3	Reps	Week 4	Reps
Standing Rotational Throw w/Band		2x6 Ea.		2x6 Ea.		2x6 Ea.		2x6 Ea.
Side Plank from Knees w/Abd.		2x5 Ea.		2x6 Ea.		2x5 Ea.		2x6 Ea.
Lateral Lunge w/Step		2x6 Ea.		2x6 Ea.		2x6 Ea.		2x6 Ea.
Single Leg Balance w/Alt. Reach		2x15 Sec. Ea.		2x15 Sec. Ea.		2x15 Sec. Ea.		2x15 Sec. Ea.

Day 1 - Lower Body Workout

	Week 1	Reps	Week 2	Reps	Week 3	Reps	Week 4	Reps
Band OH Squat		8		8		8		8
		8		8		8		8
		8		8		8		8
Quadruped Position Band SA OH Press		8 Ea.		8 Ea.		8 Ea.		8 Ea.
		8 Ea.		8 Ea.		8 Ea.		8 Ea.
		8 Ea.		8 Ea.		8 Ea.		8 Ea.
Standing Chop or Lift w/Band (Pick One)		3x8 Ea.		3x8 Ea.		3x8 Ea.		3x8 Ea.
HK Band Vertical Pulldown		12		12		12		12
		12		12		12		12
		12		12		12		12
Band Split Stance SL RDL 3 Sec. Eccentric		8 Ea.		8 Ea.		8 Ea.		8 Ea.
		8 Ea.		8 Ea.		8 Ea.		8 Ea.
		8 Ea.		8 Ea.		8 Ea.		8 Ea.
Calf Raise w/3 Sec. Eccentric		3x8 Ea.		3x8 Ea.		3x8 Ea.		3x8 Ea.

Day 2 - Upper Body Workout

	Week 1	Reps	Week 2	Reps	Week 3	Reps	Week 4	Reps
Band RDL w/3 Sec. Eccentric		10		10		10		10
		10		10		10		10
		10		10		10		10
Band Row		8 Ea.		8 Ea.		8 Ea.		8 Ea.
		8 Ea.		8 Ea.		8 Ea.		8 Ea.
		8 Ea.		8 Ea.		8 Ea.		8 Ea.
Band Pullaparts (Optional: Single Arm)		3x10 Ea.		3x10 Ea.		3x10 Ea.		3x10 Ea.
Standing SA Press		8 Ea.		8 Ea.		8 Ea.		8 Ea.
		8 Ea.		8 Ea.		8 Ea.		8 Ea.
		8 Ea.		8 Ea.		8 Ea.		8 Ea.
Goblet Split Squat w/Band		8 Ea.		8 Ea.		8 Ea.		8 Ea.
		8 Ea.		8 Ea.		8 Ea.		8 Ea.
		8 Ea.		8 Ea.		8 Ea.		8 Ea.
Standing Calf Raise		3x8 Ea.		3x8 Ea.		3x8 Ea.		3x8 Ea.

Day 1 - Conditioning: Bikes, Running, or Walking - :15 Seconds Fast/:30 Seconds Rest or Slow [Week - 1 (x8), 2, (x8), 3 (x10), 4 (x10)]

Day 2 - Conditioning: Super Speed Sticks (Phase 2 - See Conditioning Section in Book for Details)

Name:

12 Week Progressive Golf Performance Program

Two Day - Phase 3

Goals:

1.) Build A Foundation of Strength

Warm-Up Mobility	Reps
Hip Flexion/Extension: Toe Touches	1x8
Hip Internal/External: Standing Hip Circles or Stork Turns	1x5 Ea.
Lower Back: Standing Pelvic Tilts	1x8 Ea.
T-Spine: A-Frame Stretch or Bent Over T-Spine External Rotations	1x8 Ea.
Scapula: Standing Wall Slides or Arm Raise w/Golf Club + Standing Arm Reaches	1x8
Shoulder: Tom House Arm Circle Circuit (6 positions: Small, Medium, Big - both forward and backwards)	10 Sec. Ea. Position
Wrist/Elbow: Power 3 w/Golf Club (Pronation & Supination + Ulnar & Radial Deviation+ Wrist Extension & Flexion)	1x6 Ea.
Neck: Standing Neck Circles	1x3 Ea.

Foam Roll	Reps
Ankle: Standing Ankle Mobs + Leg Swings	1x8 Ea.
Knee: Standing Quad Pull w/Straight Leg + Standing Single Leg Hip Flexion	5 Sec. Holds (x2 Ea. Side)

Day 1 - Warm-Up Circuit	Week 1	Reps	Week 2	Reps	Week 3	Reps	Week 4	Reps
Single Leg Jump Squat		2x8 Ea.		2x8 Ea.		2x8 Ea.		2x8 Ea.
Long Lever Plank		2x8 Br.		2x8 Br.		2x8 Br.		2x8 Br.
SL Bucks		2x8 Ea.		2x8 Ea.		2x8 Ea.		2x8 Ea.
Bird Dogs w/No Feet		2x6 Ea.		2x6 Ea.		2x6 Ea.		2x6 Ea.

Day 2 - Warm-Up Circuit	Week 1	Reps	Week 2	Reps	Week 3	Reps	Week 4	Reps
Stepping Rotational Throw w/Band		2x6 Ea.		2x6 Ea.		2x6 Ea.		2x6 Ea.
Side plank		2x8 Ea.		2x8 Ea.		2x8 Ea.		2x8 Ea.
Lateral Lunge Band Pressout		2x6 Ea.		2x6 Ea.		2x6 Ea.		2x6 Ea.
Single Leg Balance w/Rotation		2x15 Sec. Ea.		2x15 Sec. Ea.		2x15 Sec. Ea.		2x15 Sec. Ea.

Day 1 - Lower Body Workout	Week 1	Reps	Week 2	Reps	Week 3	Reps	Week 4	Reps
OH Squat w/Pause		8		8		8		8
		8		8		8		8
		8		8		8		8
Pushup Hold w/Band SA OH Press		8 Ea.		8 Ea.		8 Ea.		8 Ea.
		8 Ea.		8 Ea.		8 Ea.		8 Ea.
		8 Ea.		8 Ea.		8 Ea.		8 Ea.
Speed Chop or Lift w/Band (Pick One)		3x8 Ea.		3x8 Ea.		3x8 Ea.		3x8 Ea.
HK Speed Vertical Pulldown		12		12		12		12
		12		12		12		12
		12		12		12		12
Band Split Stance SL RDL w/Speed		8 Ea.		8 Ea.		8 Ea.		8 Ea.
		8 Ea.		8 Ea.		8 Ea.		8 Ea.
		8 Ea.		8 Ea.		8 Ea.		8 Ea.
Single Leg Calf Raise w/Single Leg Eccentric		3x8 Ea.		3x8 Ea.		3x8 Ea.		3x8 Ea.

Day 2 - Upper Body Workout	Week 1	Reps	Week 2	Reps	Week 3	Reps	Week 4	Reps
Band RDL w/Speed		10		10		10		10
		10		10		10		10
		10		10		10		10
Band Row w/Speed		8 Ea.		8 Ea.		8 Ea.		8 Ea.
		8 Ea.		8 Ea.		8 Ea.		8 Ea.
		8 Ea.		8 Ea.		8 Ea.		8 Ea.
Band Pullaparts + No Money's (Optional: Single Arm)		3x10 Ea.		3x10 Ea.		3x10 Ea.		3x10 Ea.
SA SL Press		12 Ea.		12 Ea.		12 Ea.		12 Ea.
		12 Ea.		12 Ea.		12 Ea.		12 Ea.
		12 Ea.		12 Ea.		12 Ea.		12 Ea.
RFE Split Squat w/Band Opt.		8 Ea.		8 Ea.		8 Ea.		8 Ea.
		8 Ea.		8 Ea.		8 Ea.		8 Ea.
		8 Ea.		8 Ea.		8 Ea.		8 Ea.
SL Standing Calf Raises		3x8 Ea.		3x8 Ea.		3x8 Ea.		3x8 Ea.

Day 1 - Conditioning: Bikes, Running, or Walking - :10 Seconds Fast/:20 Seconds Rest or Slow [Week - 1 (x10), 2, (x10), 3 (x12), 4 (x12)]

Day 2 - Conditioning: Super Speed Sticks (Phase 2 - See Conditioning Section in Book for Details)

Name:

12 Week Progressive Golf Performance Program

Four Day - Phase 1

Goals:

1.) Build A Foundation of Strength

Foam Roll:

Mobility	Reps
Ankle: Supine Ankle Flexion & Extension + Supine Ankle Windshield Wipers	1x8 Ea.
Knee: Supine Knee Flexion/Extension	5 Sec. Holds (x2 Ea. Side)
Hip Extension/Flexion: Alt. Leg Lowers	1x8 Ea.
Hip Internal/External: Supine Hip Circles or Passive Straight Leg Twist	1x5 Ea.
Lower Back: Supine Pelvic Tilts	1x8 Ea.
T-Spine: Supine Arm Bar (Progression: Add a Kettlebell or Dumbbell)	1x8 Ea.
Scapula: Supine Floor Slides + Supine Arm Reaches	1x6 Ea.
Shoulder: *Targeted Above in a Two-in-One Exercises - Supine Arm Bar w/Internal and External Rotation (Progression: Add a Kettlebell or Dumbbell)	
Wrist/Elbow: Supine Wrist Press Ups + Ulnar and Radial Wrist Flexion + Supine Wrist Flexion and Extension	1x6 Ea.
Neck: Supine Neck Flexion & Extension + Supine Neck Side to Side Rotations	1x3 Ea.

Day 1 & 3 - Warm-Up Circuit:	Week 1	Reps	Week 2	Reps	Week 3	Reps	Week 4	Reps
Jump Squats		2x8		2x8		2x8		2x8
Push-Up Hold		2x8 Br.		2x8 Br.		2x8 Br.		2x8 Br.
SL Cook Hip Lift		2x8 Ea.		2x8 Ea.		2x8 Ea.		2x8 Ea.
Bird Dogs		2x6 Ea.		2x6 Ea.		2x6 Ea.		2x6 Ea.

Day 2 & 4 - Warm-Up Circuit:	Week 1	Reps	Week 2	Reps	Week 3	Reps	Week 4	Reps
Half-Kneeling Rotational Throw w/Band		2x6 Ea.		2x6 Ea.		2x6 Ea.		2x6 Ea.
Side Plank from Knees		2x8 Ea.		2x8 Ea.		2x8 Ea.		2x8 Ea.
Assisted Lateral Lunge w/Band		2x6 Ea.		2x6 Ea.		2x6 Ea.		2x6 Ea.
Single Leg Balance		2x15 Sec. Ea.		2x15 Sec. Ea.		2x15 Sec. Ea.		2x15 Sec. Ea.

Day 1 - Lower Body Workout	Week 1	Reps	Week 2	Reps	Week 3	Reps	Week 4	Reps
Goblet Split Squat w/Band on Inside or Outside of Knee		8 Ea.		8 Ea.		8 Ea.		8 Ea.
		8 Ea.		8 Ea.		8 Ea.		8 Ea.
		8 Ea.		8 Ea.		8 Ea.		8 Ea.
Band RDL		10		10		10		10
		10		10		10		10
		10		10		10		10
HK Anti-Rotation Press		3x8 Ea.		3x8 Ea.		3x8 Ea.		3x8 Ea.
Seated Calf Raise w/Band		3x8 Ea.		3x8 Ea.		3x8 Ea.		3x8 Ea.

Day 2 - Upper Body Workout	Week 1	Reps	Week 2	Reps	Week 3	Reps	Week 4	Reps
Quadruped w/Band Eccentric OH Press		8 Ea.		8 Ea.		8 Ea.		8 Ea.
		8 Ea.		8 Ea.		8 Ea.		8 Ea.
		8 Ea.		8 Ea.		8 Ea.		8 Ea.
Band Row w/Pause		8 Ea.		8 Ea.		8 Ea.		8 Ea.
		8 Ea.		8 Ea.		8 Ea.		8 Ea.
		8 Ea.		8 Ea.		8 Ea.		8 Ea.
HK Lift w/Band		3x8 Ea.		3x8 Ea.		3x8 Ea.		3x8 Ea.
Band No Money's (Optional: Single Arm)		3x10 Ea.		3x10 Ea.		3x10 Ea.		3x10 Ea.

Day 3 - Lower Body Workout	Week 1	Reps	Week 2	Reps	Week 3	Reps	Week 4	Reps
Goblet Squat w/BAK		8		8		8		8
		8		8		8		8
		8		8		8		8
Band Split Stance SL RDL		8 Ea.		8 Ea.		8 Ea.		8 Ea.
		8 Ea.		8 Ea.		8 Ea.		8 Ea.
		8 Ea.		8 Ea.		8 Ea.		8 Ea.
HK Anti-Lateral Flexion		3x8 Ea.		3x8 Ea.		3x8 Ea.		3x8 Ea.
Seated Tib Anterior		3x8 Ea.		3x8 Ea.		3x8 Ea.		3x8 Ea.

Day 4 - Upper Body Workout	Week 1	Reps	Week 2	Reps	Week 3	Reps	Week 4	Reps
HK SA Press		8 Ea.		8 Ea.		8 Ea.		8 Ea.
		8 Ea.		8 Ea.		8 Ea.		8 Ea.
		8 Ea.		8 Ea.		8 Ea.		8 Ea.
HK SA Band Vertical Pulldown		8 Ea.		8 Ea.		8 Ea.		8 Ea.
		8 Ea.		8 Ea.		8 Ea.		8 Ea.
		8 Ea.		8 Ea.		8 Ea.		8 Ea.
HK Chop w/Band		3x8 Ea.		3x8 Ea.		3x8 Ea.		3x8 Ea.
Band No Money's (Optional: Single Arm)		3x10 Ea.		3x10 Ea.		3x10 Ea.		3x10 Ea.

Day 1 & 3 - Conditioning: Bikes, Running, or Walking - :30 Seconds Medium-Fast/:30 Seconds Rest or Slow [Week - 1 (x6), 2, (x6), 3 (x8), 4 (x8)]

Day 2 & 4 - Conditioning: Super Speed Sticks (Phase 1 - See Conditioning Section in Book for Details)

Days 1 & 3

Name:								
12 Week Progressive Golf Performance Program								
Four Day - Phase 2								
Goals:								
1.) Build A Foundation of Strength								
Foam Roll:		Reps						
Ankle: HK Ankle Dorso-Flexion + HK Side to Side Ankle Dorso-Flexion		1x8 Ea.						
Knee: Quadruped Single Leg Extension		1x8 Ea.						

Day 1 & 3 - Warm-Up Circuit:	Week 1	Reps	Week 2	Reps	Week 3	Reps	Week 4	Reps
Single Leg Jump Squat w/Bilateral Landing		2x4 Ea.		2x4 Ea.		2x4 Ea.		2x4 Ea.
Plank		2x8 Br.		2x8 Br.		2x8 Br.		2x8 Br.
SL Cook Hip Lift w/Hold (10 Sec.)		2x3 Ea.		2x3 Ea.		2x3 Ea.		2x3 Ea.
Bird Dogs Holds (5 Sec. Ea.)		2x3 Ea.		2x3 Ea.		2x3 Ea.		2x3 Ea.
Day 1 - Lower Body Workout	Week 1	Reps	Week 2	Reps	Week 3	Reps	Week 4	Reps
Goblet Split Squat w/Band		8 Ea.		8 Ea.		8 Ea.		8 Ea.
		8 Ea.		8 Ea.		8 Ea.		8 Ea.
		8 Ea.		8 Ea.		8 Ea.		8 Ea.
Band RDL w/Eccentric		10		10		10		10
		10		10		10		10
		10		10		10		10
Anti-Rotation Press w/Hold (15 Sec.)		x3 Ea.		x3 Ea.		x3 Ea.		x3 Ea.
Standing Calf Raise		3x8 Ea.		3x8 Ea.		3x8 Ea.		3x8 Ea.
Day 3 - Lower Body Workout	Week 1	Reps	Week 2	Reps	Week 3	Reps	Week 4	Reps
Band OH Squat		8		8		8		8
		8		8		8		8
		8		8		8		8
Band Split Stance SL RDL 3 Sec. Eccentric		8 Ea.		8 Ea.		8 Ea.		8 Ea.
		8 Ea.		8 Ea.		8 Ea.		8 Ea.
		8 Ea.		8 Ea.		8 Ea.		8 Ea.
Isometric Anti-Lateral Flexion		3x8 Ea.		3x8 Ea.		3x8 Ea.		3x8 Ea.
Standing Calf Raise w/3 Sec. Eccentric		3x8 Ea.		3x8 Ea.		3x8 Ea.		3x8 Ea.

Day 1 & 3 - Conditioning: Bikes, Running, or Walking - :15 Seconds Fast/:30 Seconds Rest or Slow [Week - 1 (x8), 2, (x8), 3 (x10), 4 (x10)]

Days 2 & 4

Hip Flexion/Extension: Quadruped Hip Extension							1x8 Ea.	
Hip Internal/External: Quadruped Hip Circles							1x6 Ea.	
Lower Back: Cat & Camels							1x8 Ea.	
T-Spine: Quadruped T-Spine Ext. Rotation (Progression: HK T-Spine Rotations)							1x8 Ea.	
Scapula: Half-Kneeling Single Arm Reach + Half-Kneeling Elevation and Depression							1x6 Ea.	
Shoulder: Half-Kneeling Arm Circle (Both forward and backward)							1x3 Ea.	
Wrist/Elbow: Quadruped Wrist Mobs (Flexion & Extension)							1x6 Ea.	
Neck: Quadruped Side to Side w/Chin to Sternum or Tall-Kneeling Side to Side Twist w/Chin to Sternum							1x3 Ea.	

Day 2 & 4 - Warm-Up Circuit:	Week 1	Reps	Week 2	Reps	Week 3	Reps	Week 4	Reps
Standing Rotational Throw w/Band		2x6 Ea.		2x6 Ea.		2x6 Ea.		2x6 Ea.
Side Plank from Knees w/Abd.		2x5 Ea.		2x5 Ea.		2x5 Ea.		2x5 Ea.
Lateral Lunge w/Step		2x6 Ea.		2x6 Ea.		2x6 Ea.		2x6 Ea.
Single Leg Balance w/Alt. Reach		2x15 Sec. Ea.		2x15 Sec. Ea.		2x15 Sec. Ea.		2x15 Sec. Ea.
Day 2 - Upper Body Workout	Week 1	Reps	Week 2	Reps	Week 3	Reps	Week 4	Reps
Quadruped Position Band SA OH Press		8 Ea.		8 Ea.		8 Ea.		8 Ea.
		8 Ea.		8 Ea.		8 Ea.		8 Ea.
		8 Ea.		8 Ea.		8 Ea.		8 Ea.
Band Row		8 Ea.		8 Ea.		8 Ea.		8 Ea.
		8 Ea.		8 Ea.		8 Ea.		8 Ea.
		8 Ea.		8 Ea.		8 Ea.		8 Ea.
Standing Lift w/Band		3x8 Ea.		3x8 Ea.		3x8 Ea.		3x8 Ea.
Band Pullaparts (Optional: Single Arm)		3x10 Ea.		3x10 Ea.		3x10 Ea.		3x10 Ea.
Day 4 - Upper Body Workout	Week 1	Reps	Week 2	Reps	Week 3	Reps	Week 4	Reps
Standing SA Press		8 Ea.		8 Ea.		8 Ea.		8 Ea.
		8 Ea.		8 Ea.		8 Ea.		8 Ea.
		8 Ea.		8 Ea.		8 Ea.		8 Ea.
HK Band Vertical Pulldown		12		12		12		12
		12		12		12		12
		12		12		12		12
Standing Chop w/Band		3x8 Ea.		3x8 Ea.		3x8 Ea.		3x8 Ea.
Band Pullaparts (Optional: Single Arm)		3x10 Ea.		3x10 Ea.		3x10 Ea.		3x10 Ea.

Day 2 & 4 - Conditioning: Super Speed Sticks (Phase 2 - See Conditioning Section in Book for Details)

Day 1 & 3	Week 1	Reps	Week 2	Reps	Week 3	Reps	Week 4	Reps	Day 2 & 4	Week 1	Reps	Week 2	Reps	Week 3	Reps	Week 4	Reps
Name:									Hip Flexion/Extension: Toe Touches		1x8						
12 Week Progressive Golf Performance Program									Hip Internal/External: Standing Hip Circles or Stork Turns		1x5 Ea.						
Four Day - Phase 3									Lower Back: Standing Pelvic Tilts		1x8 Ea.						
Goals:									T-Spine: A-Frame Stretch or Bent Over T-Spine External Rotations		1x8 Ea.						
1.) Build A Foundation of Strength									Scapula: Standing Wall Slides or Arm Raise w/Golf Club + Standing Arm Reaches		1x8						
Foam Roll:		Reps							Shoulder: Tom House Arm Circle Circuit (6 positions: Small, Medium, Big - both forward and backwards)		10 Sec. Ea. Position						
Ankle: Standing Ankle Mobs + Leg Swings		1x8 Ea.							Wrist/Elbow: Power 3 w/Golf Club (Pronation & Supination + Ulnar & Radial Deviation + Wrist Extension & Flexion)		1x6 Ea.						
Knee: Standing Active Hip Flexion and Extension		5 Sec. Holds (x2 Ea. Side)							Neck: Standing Neck Circles		1x3 Ea.						
Day 1 & 3 - Warm-Up Circuit:	Week 1	Reps	Week 2	Reps	Week 3	Reps	Week 4	Reps	Day 2 & 4 - Warm-Up Circuit:	Week 1	Reps	Week 2	Reps	Week 3	Reps	Week 4	Reps
Single Leg Jump Squat		2x8 Ea.		2x8 Ea.		2x8 Ea.		2x8 Ea.	Stepping Rotational Throw w/Band		2x6 Ea.		2x6 Ea.		2x6 Ea.		2x6 Ea.
Long Lever Plank		2x8 Br.		2x8 Br.		2x8 Br.		2x8 Br.	Side plank		2x8 Ea.		2x8 Ea.		2x8 Ea.		2x8 Ea.
SL Bucks		2x8 Ea.		2x8 Ea.		2x8 Ea.		2x8 Ea.	Lateral Lunge Band Pressout		2x6 Ea.		2x6 Ea.		2x6 Ea.		2x6 Ea.
Bird Dogs w/No Feet		2x6 Ea.		2x6 Ea.		2x6 Ea.		2x6 Ea.	Single Leg Balance w/Rotation		2x15 Sec. Ea.		2x15 Sec. Ea.		2x15 Sec. Ea.		2x15 Sec. Ea.
Day 1 - Lower Body Workout	Week 1	Reps	Week 2	Reps	Week 3	Reps	Week 4	Reps	Day 2 - Upper Body Workout	Week 1	Reps	Week 2	Reps	Week 3	Reps	Week 4	Reps
RFE Split Squat w/Band Optional		8 Ea.		8 Ea.		8 Ea.		8 Ea.	Pushup Hold w/Band SA OH Press		8 Ea.		8 Ea.		8 Ea.		8 Ea.
		8 Ea.		8 Ea.		8 Ea.		8 Ea.			8 Ea.		8 Ea.		8 Ea.		8 Ea.
		8 Ea.		8 Ea.		8 Ea.		8 Ea.			8 Ea.		8 Ea.		8 Ea.		8 Ea.
Band RDL w/Speed		10		10		10		10	Band Row w/Speed		8 Ea.		8 Ea.		8 Ea.		8 Ea.
		10		10		10		10			8 Ea.		8 Ea.		8 Ea.		8 Ea.
		10		10		10		10			8 Ea.		8 Ea.		8 Ea.		8 Ea.
Standing Anti-Rotation Press		3x8 Ea.		3x8 Ea.		3x8 Ea.		3x8 Ea.	Speed Lift w/Band		3x8 Ea.		3x8 Ea.		3x8 Ea.		3x8 Ea.
Standing SL Calf Raise		3x8 Ea.		3x8 Ea.		3x8 Ea.		3x8 Ea.	Band Pullaparts + No Money's (Optional: Single Arm)		3x10 Ea.		3x10 Ea.		3x10 Ea.		3x10 Ea.
Day 3 - Lower Body Workout	Week 1	Reps	Week 2	Reps	Week 3	Reps	Week 4	Reps	Day 4 - Upper Body Workout	Week 1	Reps	Week 2	Reps	Week 3	Reps	Week 4	Reps
Band OH Squat w/Pause		8		8		8		8	SA SL Press		12 Ea.		12 Ea.		12 Ea.		12 Ea.
		8		8		8		8			12 Ea.		12 Ea.		12 Ea.		12 Ea.
		8		8		8		8			12 Ea.		12 Ea.		12 Ea.		12 Ea.
Band Split Stance SL RDL w/Speed		8 Ea.		8 Ea.		8 Ea.		8 Ea.	HK Speed Vertical Pulldown		12		12		12		12
		8 Ea.		8 Ea.		8 Ea.		8 Ea.			12		12		12		12
		8 Ea.		8 Ea.		8 Ea.		8 Ea.			12		12		12		12
Standing Anti-Lateral Flexion		3x8 Ea.		3x8 Ea.		3x8 Ea.		3x8 Ea.	Speed Chop w/Band		3x8 Ea.		3x8 Ea.		3x8 Ea.		3x8 Ea.
Single Leg Calf Raise w/Single Leg Eccentric		3x8 Ea.		3x8 Ea.		3x8 Ea.		3x8 Ea.	Band Pullaparts + No Money's (Optional: Single Arm)		3x10 Ea.		3x10 Ea.		3x10 Ea.		3x10 Ea.
Day 1 & 3 - Conditioning: Bikes, Running, or Walking - :10 Seconds Fast/:20 Seconds Rest or Slow [Week - 1 (x10), 2, (x10), 3 (x12), 4 (x12)]									Day 2 & 4 - Conditioning: Super Speed Sticks (Phase 2 - See Conditioning Section in Book for Details)								

Giving Credit Where It's Due

It's always important to give credit where it's due and I want to thank many of the mentors who have helped me out along the way.

Randy Myers (Sea Island, GA)

During a 15-minute phone call when I was 20 years old, Randy told me everything I needed to do to succeed as an elite golf fitness professional. He pushed me to work harder and helped me pave a path for success in the golf fitness industry.

Alex Merrill (Raleigh, NC)

Alex is one of the best mentors I have ever had. He taught me how to individualize programs in a group setting, how to work alongside with swing/golf coaches, and he also helped pave a path for me in the golf fitness industry in more ways than he knows.

David Donatucci (Palm Beach Gardens, FL) & Barrett Stover (Orlando, FL)

I spent seven months shadowing and helping Dave and Barrett at the Florida Institute of Performance in Palm Beach Gardens, FL. This opportunity allowed me to see what it was like to work with some of the top PGA and LPGA Tour players in the world. They consistently challenged me to continue my education, to keep learning; they were the main reason I got my Master's Degree in Exercise Science.

The Team at Mike Boyle Strength & Conditioning (Woburn, MA)

This is one of the most elite facilities that I have ever seen and was fortunate enough to have the opportunity to intern there for 3 months. The environment at Mike Boyle Strength & Conditioning is positive, informative, and very detailed. The staff and athletes are incredible there.

Brendon Rearick (San Jose, CA) & Kevin Carr (Boston, MA)

Brendon and Kevin were my internship directors during my time at Mike Boyle Strength & Conditioning. They have continued to give me advice over the last 5 years to keep pushing me forward in the right direction to be a better coach and overall person.

Mike Manavian (Greenwich, CT)

Mike has taught me the passion that is needed to be able to write a book, the work ethic that it takes to be elite at whatever it is you do, and he always keeps me on my toes.

Ali Gilbert (Greenwich, CT)

Ali has pushed me to be better in multiple ways. She has consistently pushed me to stay open-minded and to keep continuing my education in a variety of ways. Specifically, with nutrition, business, personal training, and public speaking.

Mike Autore (New York, NY)

Spending just over two years working under Mike led to many positives attributes that rubbed off on me. Mike's ability to relate to and understand people is like no other. He continually pushed me to train and work harder, but also to have fun while doing it.

Charlie Weingroff (Greenwich, CT)

I have been attending Charlie's seminars/speeches since 2014. A major reason that I was able to write this book was due to the basic principles that Charlie has preached about throughout his various presentations.

Jerry Hogge & The Entire Golf Staff at Methodist University (Fayetteville, NC)

Mr. Hogge taught me the importance of reading and how much you can benefit from it. The opportunities he gave and taught me are a major reason why this book has been able to be put together. The entire golf staff at MU has supported me in various ways and I can't thank them enough for their help along the way.

Robert Fritz (Greensboro, NC)

Robbie is one of my most influential golf mentors. He is someone who consistently tries to improve as a swing instructor and in life in general. After taking dozens and dozens of lessons from him, I will stick to my word in saying that he is one of the best golf instructors in the world.

Chris Finn (Morrisville, NC)

I've been learning from Chris since my senior year of college. Chris has taught me to dream big, the importance of backing up workout plans with research, and has been a great mentor who always seems to overdeliver.

Andy Frisella (St. Louis, MO)

This book probably would not have been written if it wasn't for the "Winning the Day Formula" that Andy taught me and preaches about in his seminars. I was fortunate enough to meet Andy in person this year to thank him.

Johnathan Fader (New York, NY)

This is a guy who I have only seen speak once and have never met. However, he taught me the importance of working on your mindset daily. Having the correct mindset was essential towards being able to have the discipline and patience to write this book.

SuperFlex Fitness and The Team at SuperSpeed Golf

Both of these companies have been very supportive and I cannot thank them enough for setting up links and discounts for the equipment needed in the 12-Week Program.

The Entire Functional Movement Screen Team

Gray Cook, Lee Burton, and Greg Rose have been key toward my development as a golf fitness professional. The FMS screen is something that I use for screening clients and has helped simplify strength and conditioning for me.

My Parents, Sister, and Brother

They are always willing to lend a hand and give advice when needed. I cannot thank them enough for their help and support.

References

1. Alvarez, M., Sedano, S., Cuadrado, G., & Redondo, J. C. (2012). Effects of an 18-week strength training program on low-handicap golfers' performance. *Journal of Strength and Conditioning Research, 26*(4), 111-1121.

2. Boyle, M. (2010). Advances in Functional Training: Training Techniques for Coaches, Personal Trainers and Athletes. *On Target Publications,* 31-34.

3. Cook, G., Burton, L, Kiesel, K., Rose, G., Bryant, M. (2010). Movement - Functional Movement Systems: Screening, Assessment and Corrective Strategies. *On Target Publications,* 323-329.

4. Doan, B. K., Newton, R. U., Kwon, Y., & Kraemer, W. J. (2006). Effects of physical conditioning on intercollegiate golfer performance. *Journal of Strength*

5. Fletcher, I. M., & Hartwell, M. (2004). Effect of an 8-week combined weights and plyometrics training program on golf drive performance. *Journal of Strength and Conditioning Research*, 18, 59–62.

6. Fradkin, A. J., Sherman, C. A., & Finch, C. F. (2004). Improving golf performance with a warm up conditioning program. *British Journal of Sports Medicine*, 38, 762–765.

7. Glass, J. (2015). Advanced Screening: How I Use The TPI Screen. http://www.mytpi.com/articles/fitness/advanced_screen ing_how_i_use_the_tpi_screen

8. Haff, G., Triplett, T. (2016). ESSENTIALS of STRENGTH TRAINING and CONDITIONING: Forth Edition. *Human Kinetics*, 8-9.

9. Hegedus, E. J., Hardesty, K. W., Sunderland, K. L., Hegedus, R. J., & Smoliga, J. M. (2016). A randomized trial of traditional and golf-specific resistance training in amateur female golfers: Benefits beyond golf performance. *Physical Therapy in Sport, 22*, 41-53.

10. Hetu, F. E., Christie, C. A., & Faigenbaum, A. D. (1998). Effects of conditioning on physical fitness and club head speed in mature golfers. *Perceptual and Motor Skills*, 86, 811–815.

11. Kim, K. J. (2010). Effects of Core Muscle Strengthening Training on Flexibility, Muscular Strength and Driver Shot Performance in Female Professional Golfers. *International Journal of Applied Sports Sciences*, 22(1), 111-127.

12. Landford J. (1976) The effect of strength training on distance and accuracy in golf. *Doctoral thesis. Brigham Young University*, 1-85.

13. Lephart, S. M., Smoliga, J. M., Myers, J. B., Sell, T. C., & Tsai, Y. (2007). An eight-week golf-specific exercise program improves physical characteristics, swing mechanics, and golf performance in recreational golfers. *Journal of Strength and Conditioning Research*, 21, 860–869.

14. Thompson, C. J., Cobb, K. M., & Blackwell, J. (2007). Functional training improves clubhead speed and functional fitness in older golfers. *Journal of Strength and Conditioning Research*, *21*(1), 131-137.

15. Sell, T. C., Tsai, Y., Smoliga, J. M., Myers, J.B., & Lephart, S. M. (2007). Strength, flexibility, and balance characteristics of highly proficient golfers. *Journal of Strength and Conditioning Research*, 21, 1166–1171.

16. Smith, C. J., Callister, R., & Lubans, D. R. (2011). A systematic review of strength and conditioning programmes designed to improve fitness characteristics in golfers. *Journal of Sports Sciences*, 29 (9), 933 –943

17. Smith, A. C., Roberts, J. R., Wallace, E. S., Pui, K., & Forrester, S. E. (2016). Comparison of Two- and Three-Dimensional Methods for Analysis of Trunk Kinematic Variables in the Golf Swing. *Journal of Applied Biomechanics*, *32*(1), 23-31.

18. Zech, A., Hübscher, M., Vogt, L., Banzer, W., Hänsel, F., & Pfeifer, K. (2010). Balance Training for Neuromuscular Control and Performance Enhancement: A Systematic Review. *Journal of Athletic Training*, *45*(4), 392–403. http://doi.org/10.4085/1062-6050-45.4.392

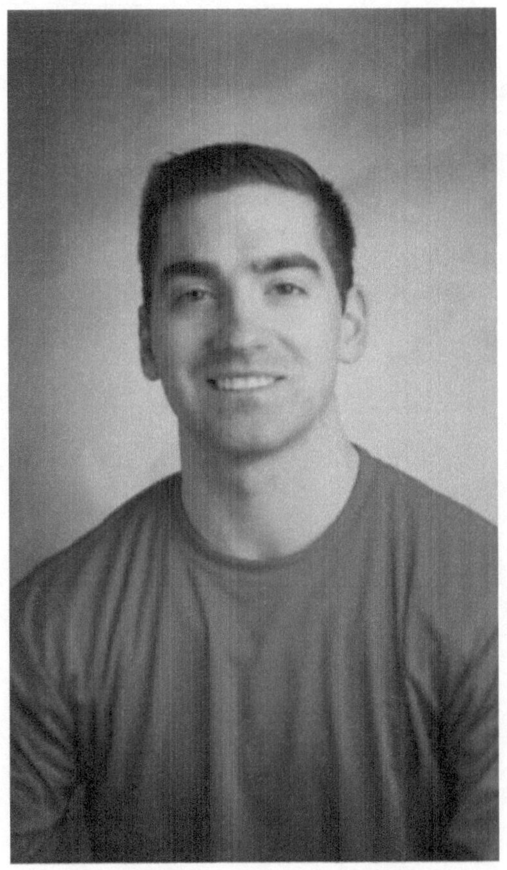

<u>A Note From the Author</u>

Thank you for reading this book and for all of the support. I wish you the best on your golf and fitness journey!